THE OVEREATING HABIT
How To Break It Using The Law of Detachment

WILLIAM F. MCLAUGHLIN

The Overeating Habit
How To Break It Using The Law of Detachment

© Copyright 2018, William F. McLaughlin.
All Rights Reserved. No part of this book may be reproduced or transmitted in any form without written permission of the publisher, except that brief passages may be quoted for reviews.

ISBN: 1720550247
ISBN-13: 978-1720550242

CoachMcLaughlin.com
Info@CoachMcLaughlin.com

**The Law of Detachment
Weight Loss Poem**

*"I enjoy five meals per day,
Eating in a slow and detached way;
Watching for the hunger to subside,
Then stopping for that is my guide!"*

CONTENTS

INTRODUCTION:
THE HABIT & THE REMEDY

The Root Cause of Overeating

The premise of this book, is that the persistently overweight person *habitually eats for emotional comfort instead of physical nourishment.* This wrong purpose and wrong relationship with food results in the virtual inability to control one's appetite, and is the root cause of overeating. What happens is this: The sensual pleasure of food overrides or masks the emotional discomfort that we bring to the table – the discomfort of stress, boredom, worry, depression, loneliness, anger, etc. Thus this seeming palliative is not only false, it's also only temporary, because soon after you stop eating the discomfort returns, doesn't it? Then all you can think about is when your next meal will be. This is no way to eat, no way to live, and is a habit that can be broken by changing your relationship both with your food – and with yourself.

The Law of Detachment Remedy

This deeply entrenched habit is broken by learning to eat *without* emotional involvement. It's learning to eat *sensually* not emotionally. It's to separate or *detach* yourself from your feelings while you're eating. You want to eat *only* with the five senses and your higher awareness – nothing else. Experience every moment and nuance of the eating process from a conscious *distance,* as if you're an outside observer or witness watching yourself eat. You want to experience eating *objectively* as well as subjectively – experience it from the outside in as well as the inside out.

When you eat in this consciously detached way, an amazing thing happens: *You become totally satisfied on a small fraction of your usual meal size!* Pounds drop on their own, naturally, without "dieting," pills or willpower.

The *law of detachment* is not new; it's as old as humanity itself. It's the very method and mindset of higher intelligence, power and freedom. It was taught by the greatest teachers in history. Take, for example, the saying of one of them, "Be in the world but not of the world." We could paraphrase it, "Be in your food but not of your food, " or "Be in your body but not of your body, " or "Eat to live; don't live to eat." And the essential teaching of another master was "the extinction of all attachment," – because, whatever you're attached to, controls you; whatever you're detached from, *you* control. This is the definition of freedom, and is the prerequisite to optimal health and happiness.

What *is* new, is that you'll be applying this universal law to achieve a specific, practical purpose – overcoming your *eating-for-comfort habit.* You're going to learn to cease being unconsciously driven by a program from the past – however acquired. You'll learn to think, feel and eat, from a conscious *distance* instead of from emotional involvement or entanglement. Living the *law of detachment* then, is the reality-based way to live a naturally healthy, happy, self-controlled life, a mind-body-spirit-controlled life. The purpose of this book is to show you how.

The Three Pillars of Natural Weight Loss

Breaking The Overeating Habit is one of three interrelated phases of your mind-body transformation. The second phase is *Revising Your Self-image* – which is about changing the way you "see" yourself, because, for the subconscious mind *perception is everything*. For example, if you "think" of yourself as overweight – even though you really are, your subconscious misinterprets this to mean that you *want* to be overweight, so will work around the clock to help keep you that way because that's how you unwittingly "programmed" it. This is one of the subtle intricacies of how the subconscious mind works – which I'll talk more about in Chapter 3, *Revising Your Self-image*.

The third overlapping phase of this unique program is *Overcoming Your Stress*. The watchword is this: Control your emotions or they'll control you – and your body. Stress is the primary trigger of your *Eating-for-Comfort Habit,* so treating it will occupy much of this book.

Applying The Law To All Experience

You'll learn to apply this law of detachment mindset not only to eating, but to all that you see, hear, think, feel and do – to clarify, control and improve every area of your life – because you don't eat with your mouth alone.

But – and this is a big but – no pun intended. In order for this natural method to work, it has to be *internalized* into your subconscious "computer." It has to *sink in* otherwise it just goes in one ear and out the other and no change happens. We'll use the power of self-hypnosis, guided meditation and visualization to impress the Method onto your subconscious mind so it becomes an integral and virtually effortless part of successful living and eating going forward.

All the chapters in this book will relate to one of these three phases.

Welcome to the greatest adventure on earth!

CHAPTER 1
THE HABIT-BREAKING METHOD

"Every battle is won before it's ever fought." – Sun Tzu

How The Habit Began

Understanding the root cause of overeating is necessary to lasting recovery. Ignorance isn't bliss; it's fattening. You don't want merely temporary, symptomatic relief. You know from painful and expensive trial and error, through diet after diet, that doesn't work. You want lasting, causal, reality-based relief. You want a natural way of being and eating you can live with, one you can "practice" for life.

How did this overeating habit arise? Why and how did you gain that excess weight in the first place? Why is it so hard to get rid of? And how can you get rid of it steadily, naturally, and without stress, strain or deprivation? In other words, you want to know what makes you tick. Socrates said, "Know thyself." When you know yourself, you know virtually everything, including how to regain control of your appetite and lose that excess weight once and for all.

All self-satisfying excuses, reasons, rationalizations and justifications aside, you're overweight because you overeat, and you overeat because you eat for the wrong reason: *You eat for emotional comfort instead of for physical nourishment.* You eat to *feel* good, and anything that makes you feel good you want more and more of it. You hate to stop eating because as soon as you do, the comfort stops too. Overeating is a habit seemingly beyond control.

This *eating-for-comfort habit* became established through no fault of your own: You acquired it during infancy from your mother's innocent practice of feeding you whenever you cried. But regardless of your and her innocense in the matter, it does remain your responsibility to break this habit, correct this erroneous program. Let's look closer at how it all started and what it consists of.

The Primal Need for Security

Our feeling safe, secure and comfortable is the foundation and primary factor motivating most all of our actions, behaviors and general pursuit of happiness. It's what drives us. We need a minimum level of security and comfort in all areas of life. We want to feel secure physically, mentally, emotionally, financially, and in our relationships with others. If we don't have this minimum level of security, we feel the negative emotions of stress, fear, depression, sadness, doubt, anxiety, worry, discontent, resentment, lack of confidence, self-esteem, etc.

Now, when you were in your mother's spa-like womb, you were as secure as one could imagine – all of your wants and needs fully and effortlessly provided for. But when you passed through the birth canal into the alien outside world, things abruptly and dramatically changed. You became the most *insecure* imaginable – from the bright lights, loud noises and cold temperature of the operating-room, from being grossly severed from mother's body, held upside down by a masked stranger and spanked till you turned purple.

There was nothing you could do but cry your heart and lungs out. You were soon returned to mother who snugly held you, gently rocked you, and then, to help comfort you, she placed a warm breast or bottle into your mouth. Having something in your mouth did stop your crying – but it contained food! And food was the last thing you wanted at the time. All you wanted was to be held and rocked – because that was the closest experience of being back in the comfort and security of your mother's womb!

Setting The Habit Via Repetition

This scenario of being fed whenever you cried was repeated hundreds of times after birth. Whenever you cried, your mother assumed either your diaper was dirty or that you were hungry. So she'd first check your diaper. If clean, she placed a breast or bottle into your mouth to feed and pacify you, and when something is put into your mouth, the instinctive reaction is to chew. But you weren't hungry all those times. Again, you just wanted to be held and rocked. The result: *You became conditioned to equate food with comfort and security!* You were innocently and inadvertently trained to eat for emotional comfort instead of for physical nourishment.

Now this wasn't much of an issue in early childhood. You were quite comfortable in your warm, cozy home with your loving parents, caring siblings and fluffy dog. But then you had to leave that comfort zone. You had to leave another secure womb. This time to attend school and relate with unfamiliar boys, girls and teachers, study difficult material, pass grueling tests and compete in rigorous sports activities. All very stressful stuff. So you reacted in the way you were trained to react in uncomfortable situations – you headed to the refrigerator for some relief.

The subtle deception about this condition is that food really *does* comfort you, but it's a falsely-based, temporary and symptomatic comfort that stops the moment you stop eating – so, you don't want to stop eating. This is not the *real* you, not the *original,* healthy, self-controlled you. You were not born to overeat, not born to eat for stress relief, not born to be powerless over food.

Understanding Powerlessness

Overeating is not a genetically-transmitted dis-ease. This overeating complex is, again, something you acquired, and regardless of how acquired, it can be dropped starting the moment you realize, with the help of your mirror and your doctor, that it's no longer serving you, that there's something wrong with this picture that you now want to correct.

That your program is *subconscious* explains why it's so difficult to stop overeating, why you feel virtually powerless over this habit, why you cannot reason yourself thinner no matter how intelligent you are, no matter how much you try. Your appeals go in one ear and out the other. The subconscious is below the level of normal awareness, out of reach of conscious, rational control. This habit continues to feel, remember and believe that food relieves your stress, so any attempt by your logical, *conscious* mind to change things is going to be stubbornly hindered or blocked.

Think of this block as a security guard complex whose job is to "protect" you by keeping you eating for the wrong reason, keeping you eating in the erroneous way it was trained. The question becomes, how do you correct this erroneous program? How do you unblock, unbrainwash this part of you? How do you reverse or neutralize this emotional attachment, this illicit love affair with food?

Breaking Your Eating-for-Comfort Habit (ECH)

You didn't overeat in a vacuum – with your mouth alone. Your thoughts, feelings and consciousness (or lack thereof) were involved as well. Effective and lasting recovery is an integrated, holistic package. To control one part of you, you have to control all parts of you. Otherwise you'd be treating the symptom, not the cause, and never reach your goal. Again, if attachment to your ECH has caused you to gain weight, then detaching from it will cause you to lose that weight. The way you reverse or neutralize the attachment is by cultivating the discipline of thinking all your thoughts, feeling all your feelings, and eating all your food, from a conscious and respectable *distance*. You think, feel and eat, not personally, but as if you were an impartial spectator, witness or outside observer.

This "distance" or space *is* the reality-based, appetite-controlling factor. It *is* the program-nullifying and neutralizing factor. You can't read a newspaper held directly against your eyes; you have to "back off" a bit in order get the clarity and power to read. You have to get as if one step removed from it.

"Keeping your distance" gives you the clarity to know when your body is satisfied along with the power to stop right then and there. You then eat only for physical nourishment and no longer for emotional nourishment. You stop eating when the body is satisfied not when the emotions are satisfied, so it becomes virtually impossible to overeat. You want to cultivate a strictly "platonic" relationship with food; that is, you want your relationship with food to be physical and sensual – *not* emotional.

Respecting the Integrity of the Relationship

The word "respectable" in this formula and context, means respecting that this is a relationship of two separate and distinct entities – your *awareness*, plus the food of which your awareness is aware. Awareness is not to be contaminated or diminished by the food the eyes are seeing, the nose is smelling, or the mouth is feeling and tasting.

Just as the ears can hear from some distance, the eyes can see from some distance, the nose can smell from some distance – *so can the mouth feel and taste from some distance!* The ears actually are *apart* from the sounds they hear, and so are the eyes, the aromas, the tastes and textures *apart* from the food being experienced. All you have to do is to *consciously* keep them that way. Keep them separate – in their correct and "lawful" relationship. That's what "keeping your distance" means and that's the primary discipline for you to practice and cultivate.

Let's look at how your mind-body-spirit faculties are related to each other and to appetite control: You have seven lower faculties and one higher faculty. The seven lower, consist of your thoughts, feelings and five-senses. The higher "spiritual" faculty is non-other than your everyday, waking *consciousness*, the part that's *aware* of the lower faculties thinking, feeling and eating. And it is by virtue of its transcendent, "above" position, that it controls your thinking, feeling and eating. You are conscious of your thoughts when you think them; therefore, your consciousness is in control of your thoughts. It's the same with your physical movements, emotional feelings, and sensual eating. Your consciousness is above them, therefore in control of them. It's your sixth sense or master sense. It's like the father/mother controlling their seven children.

Here's the problem restated: When you're eating from your "program" you're not eating from full consciousness – so there's little or no control. It's like the parent is absent and the children run wild. When eating from your program, you're eating only physically, mentally, emotionally and sensually. Your higher consciousness, your very source of clarity and power, is virtually absent from the equation, absent from the experience. You overeat because there's insufficient awareness to inform you of satiety and insufficient power to stop you.

A poem by Louisa May Alcott states the matter more succinctly:

> *"A little kingdom I possess,*
> *Where thoughts and feelings dwell;*
> *And very hard the task I find,*
> *Of governing it well."*

"Keeping your distance" brings your higher consciousness, your higher power, back into the picture, back into its correct and rightful position of supremacy over the lower faculties, back into "mind over matter." Detachment is a backward movement – away from the impotent lower, and toward the powerful higher. You become a centered personality, a centered eater.

The Three Levels of Eating Awareness

There are three levels of awareness while eating. The lowest level is virtually *unconscious* eating. That's when you eat, for example, while watching TV, reading, working, driving, etc. You're eating with so little awareness that you don't know you've had enough until it's too late, until you've overeaten by hundreds, even thousands of calories. And the worst part is, you're still hungry! It's like a big dog that swallows the whole can of food in one quick gulp, then quizzically looks up as if to say, "Is that it? Where's my meal? You call that dinner?" He's never satisfied because he never really tastes his food nor aware whether he's full. And without awareness of satiety there's also no ability to stop. Awareness is power – stopping power.

The second level of eating is *emotional* eating. Again, you eat because it seems to make you *feel* better. You eat to relax tension or stress. Again, you use food to relieve some negative emotion such as boredom, resentment, doubt, fear, uncertainty, etc. And when anything makes you feel good, you want to continue it. Not only do you not want to stop, you become hardly able to stop. You become virtually powerless over food. With unconscious eating you don't know you've had enough; with emotional eating, you not only don't know you've had enough, you don't care either; and even when you do care, you still can't stop.

Here again consciousness is virtually absent from the eating equation, leaving you without clarity and power. You're disconnected from it. Devoid of it. You're like a kitchen toaster that's not plugged into its source or power, so can't achieve its intended purpose, can't fulfill its toast-making potential. The mental faculty is *only* for thinking. The emotional faculty is *only* for feeling. The sensual, *only* for sensing. None of these lower faculties have controls of their own. They need a higher power *outside and separate* from themselves. *Detached awareness* is what gives us power over the lower faculties.

Awareness is *above* thinking, feeling and eating, so your goal and purpose here is to reach that state of "aboveness" and stay there. "Keeping your distance" is how you get above and beyond them, how you get conscious, get control, get real, get healthier, happier and slimmer.

Raising Your Level of Awareness

The third and highest level of eating is eating with full consciousness or full awareness. You may "think" you eat consciously, but consciousness comes in many degrees. If you're overweight, that's clear and incontrovertible evidence that your awareness level is low. And the way to raise awareness, again, is to get some distance or separation from the sensual eating experience. This space is necessary to clarity and power. You have to get some distance from the food in order to gain first-hand knowledge of satiety and its consequent stopping power. Detachment and consciousness are directly reciprocal: You can't be one without the other. You can't be more aware unless more detached, and vice versa.

The 3-Phase, Habit-Breaking, Appetite-Reducing, Weight-Losing Method:

EAT SLOWLY AND DETACHEDLY, WATCHING VERY INTENTLY FOR THE EXACT POINT THE HUNGER

SUBSIDES, THEN STOP!

Here's a brief outline of the three overlapping, interrelated phases:

Phase One: – is *Eating Slowly* – chewing each morsel 30 times before swallowing. You eat slowly for three essential reasons: one, to savor the food more completely; two, because it takes *time* – sometimes minutes, for the stomach to inform the brain that the body is sated; and three, to more readily identify the *exact* point or moment the body is sated.

Phase Two: – is *Eating with Detached Awareness*. Eating "from a distance" is the reality-based perspective that gives the *unprecedented clarity* to know when the body has had enough food. This clarity brings the effortless power to stop eating at will.

Detachment comes by degree with continued practice. It's not difficult in itself; it's just difficult because we're not used to it. We're used to being engrossed in our food, not above and distinct from it.

Phase Three: – is *Watching Very Attentively For The Exact Point The Hunger Subsides*. You remain hyper aware, like a Samurai warrior, for the first sense or inkling that the hunger you brought to the table has abated. Notice that you're not eating till full – *never* eating till full, because by then it's too late. If you eat till full, you'll *gain* weight not lose weight. That's the incorrect, habitual way you ate in the past.

You're eating *only until the edge has been taken off*. This happens when you've eaten about one-third to one-half of your former meal size. Sometimes the hunger abates after just a few forkfuls of food. Sometimes the hunger abates just from cooking and smelling the food – proving that your body wasn't hungry at all, or not as hungry as you "thought." Eating is not a time for thinking; it's a time for *knowing*, and the only way to know is via objective or detached awareness. The result is you'll eat less but enjoy it much more.

Then you immediately *stop eating*! Even if there's just a tiny morsel left on the plate – don't eat it because that will likely be the straw that breaks the stomach's back. Then wrap the leftovers for a future meal. – And be prepared to *always* have leftovers. A general rule of thumb is this: If you've eaten everything on your plate, you've probably overeaten.

That's it. Deceptively simple. Immensely powerful. You eat when hungry then stop when no longer hungry, but the body will stop being hungry on a small fraction of your usual meal size – because that's all it ever wanted or needed. But a little "distance" was needed to realize that weight-losing fact.

Pounds drop in due course without stress, willpower or undue feelings of deprivation. Food is no longer an issue in your life. The fact is this: *It's virtually impossible to overeat when you eat from a respectable and appropriate distance.* You know clearly when the body is sated, and you powerfully stop right then and there. Clarity and appetite-control power go hand in hand.

You're now in control of your mind and body, savoring every meal objectively, dispassionately, impersonally. You now eat like a gourmet, not like a glutton. Eating is now a meaningful, intimate experience – again, physically and sensually intimate, not *emotionally* intimate. You eat with reverence now. You eat with appreciation and gratitude now. You're not just feeding your face; you are deliciously nourishing your slimmer, healthier body. You now treat eating as a meditation. In fact, you make it a meditation – like the *Japanese Tea Ceremony*, for example, where super attention is paid to every nuance of preparing and serving a simple cup of tea – transforming the experience from mundane to sacred.

Practicing The Method At A Restaurant

If you can eat detachedly at a restaurant with its myriad distractions, you'll easily be able to eat detachedly at home. Imagine that you and two friends are entering a restaurant, perhaps one of your favorite Italian restaurants, for a nice leisurely dinner. You, of course, now try to eat *all* your meals in a leisurely rather than rushed manner regardless of whether home alone or out with others.

You use the entrance to the restaurant as a trigger for entering *detachment or hyper awareness mode*. The smiling hostess seats you at a corner booth and hands you the parchment-paper menu. You detachedly notice how elegant the crispy paper feels in your hands.

You witness the olfactory sense begin to awaken as the distinctive and attractive smell of pungent garlic permeates the room. You open the starched, white cotton napkin and place it on your lap. The impatient new waiter arrives for your order before you've even opened the menu, but it doesn't disturb you as it would've in the past. In the past you'd have carried on a diatribe in your mind about what an incompetent oaf is this waiter – then you'd proceed to eat twice as much food as planned. You quickly recover yourself because you left home *anticipating* such distractions and temptations would occur.

Sensual Awakening

You order the *Eggplant Parmigiana*. The group agrees on a bottle of *Sangiovese* wine. The eyes see a rosy pink carnation at the center of the round table and the nose smells its sweet perfume. The ears hear opera singing in the background. Sounds like Pavarotti or Boccelli. The volume is a bit too loud, though. A little disconcerting – proving you let yourself get caught up in the sound rather than remain above it. The volume should be so set that diners can tune it in or out at will. Normally you'd complain to management, but you're a different person now. You understand that resentment and judgment – all negative emotions, are fattening; all will trigger your *eating-for-comfort habit*. You accept life – and restaurants, on their terms. You let things pass now. Maintain your poise. Practice a little tongue control. Don't think anything more of it. Becoming more confident and proud of yourself now.

The ears detachedly hear the busy, quiet din of about forty other diners in the room. The ambience is relaxed and pleasant – just like you always are now – well, almost always. Progress not perfection is your watchword. The initial sounds and smells serve both as sensual appetizers and as a reminder to not allow anything to distract you from your super-conscious eating agenda.

Soon the waiter places the plate in front of you – from the wrong side of course. You pause and take a deep breath.

Then the eyes witness the entree you've chosen. You've ordered this dish many times, but now it's as if seeing it for the very first time. How visually appealing its appearance and presentation. The eyes witness the shapes and sizes of all the items – placed in so balanced and symmetrical a pattern. The eyes relish how vivid and varied the colors. It's a work of art. Just the sight of it causes salivation to begin. And you remember that it's not "you" seeing the food; it's the *eyes* seeing the food. The "you" remains above and distinct from the eyes seeing the food. And that's exactly the separation that gives you your increased clarity, power and slimmer body.

Eating Slowly and Detachedly

You then briefly close those delighted eyes and say silently but firmly to yourself the words, *slow and detached*. You open your eyes, mentally prepared to eat slowly and from a conscious *distance*. Slowly and from a *respectable* distance. You're respecting both the food and your sacred, one and only body. Everything's as if in silent, slow motion now. You're as if caught up in a reverie of present-moment super-consciousness.

The hands pick up the knife and fork noticing how heavy and nicely engraved they are. You watch the hands cut a small morsel of the steaming, mozzarella-covered eggplant. You're sure it'd be all right, etiquette-wise, to cut two pieces at a time – but that'd be contrary to your slow-eating strategy. You return the knife to the plate and transfer the fork to your right hand – purposely using the American zigzag method rather than the Continental. Though less efficient, it's more conducive to controlled, deliberate eating.

You slowly lift the eggplant straight up and into the mouth. Then you return the fork to the plate and return your hand to your knee. You don't put more food into the mouth until the previous portion has been completely chewed and swallowed. You eat this mindfully even when alone – especially when alone.

The mouth chews very, very slowly – at least thirty times, depending on the density of the food, because you know *it takes time for the stomach to inform the brain that it's had enough.* Slow it down. There's no need to rush. When you feel like giving up, remember why you held on for so long in the first place. The restaurant won't close for hours. You take twice as long to eat half as much. Your digestive system thanks you as it can now process the food easier and more efficiently. Even the lungs breathe easier. You're eating at just the right pace, at just the right rate.

Managing Your Emotions

The waiter comes over to refill the water glasses. He picks up the glasses with his fingers around the rim – where you put your mouth. What a dork! You start chewing like mad – because now you're angry. You stuff a huge forkful of linguine into your mouth, then another, then another. Your cheeks blow up like a squirrel. You soon catch yourself. You stop, take a deep breath, calm down. The old you would've carried the resentment all evening – and overeaten by a few thousand calories. You don't ever have to do that again. For the rest of the meal, you drink your water with a straw. It's settled. You're never too old to grow up.

You maintain detached attention to eating while you're talking. You can do two things at the same time. Martha asks if you've become vegetarian because of your eggplant choice. You say your definition of a vegetarian is someone who doesn't eat steak unless someone else is paying for it. Everyone laughs – but you couldn't help wondering if she was referring to you, as you're sometimes accused of being frugal to a fault.

Martha says, "I'm on a seafood diet – I see food and I eat it." The laughter continues as the waiter empties the wine bottle into their glasses.

Then Jackie says, "You know, the trouble with eating Italian food is that five or six days later, you're hungry again!"

Being Hyper Aware

You're able to maintain hyper awareness even through the laughter. The mouth gently caresses the food. The tongue moves the food from side to side and back and forth and round and round on the tongue, cheeks, palate, lips and teeth. The sharp, front incisors bite into the food, then the cuspids chew it into small pieces. The bicuspids break up and crush the course food while the multi-surfaced molars in back do most of the chewing. You want to get the very most benefit from every single morsel, to not miss the tiniest iota of delicious flavor.

The mouth is eating less but enjoying it so much more. The mouth detachedly *feels* the hot or cold temperature and the smooth and crunchy textures of the food, as thousands of happy little taste buds now burst open to begin savoring a circus of delightful flavors and aromas. You watch the mouth taste how sweet or sour, how salty or bitter, how spicy or bland, how sharp or mild, how pungent or delicate, how juicy and succulent. You *witness* the salivation and gentle swallowing as the solids become almost liquid. Mahatma Ghandi said, "You should drink your food and eat your water."

Pausing Between Bites

You stop between bites to discern whether or not the body is sated – because, again, *it takes time for the stomach to inform the brain that it's had enough.* You slowly reach over and grasp the bowl of your wine glass and lift it to the mouth.

Wine Tasting

Stopping to sip the wine or water gives you a perfect opportunity to reflect on whether the body is yet sated. You *honestly* decide it isn't. But you know very well that alcohol can and will lower inhibitions as well as awareness levels, so you're especially careful to not let it distract you.

You lift the glass to eye level and swirl it around a bit. The eyes see its brownish, mahogany color, and how fast the legs streak down the glass. You notice how the bouquet reaches the nose before the glass touches the lips. The nose sniffs the wine – first from a little distance, then you put the nose deep into the glass to notice an earthy, herbal aroma – perhaps black cherry. You've heard that taste is eighty-percent smell.

The lips pucker up, take a sip, and swirl it around in the mouth to expose it to all the taste buds. The full body, smoothness and dryness are the first impressions on the palate. The throat swallows now and you detachedly notice the remnants of the aftertaste on the back of the throat. The taste lingers to embellish the next bite of food.

While you're eating, awareness remains *undistractedly* rooted in the present moment, immediately noticing when that awareness wanders or the conversation distracts you, then you return intimate, dispassionate, platonic attention to the delicious, nourishing food. You're beginning to notice that the amount of food and drink you consume has nothing to do with quality of the dining experience. A little is a lot. You're not dulled by food and drink like the unenlightened diner; you start the meal sharp and remain so to the end of the meal.

Keeping The Eater Above the Food

You find that you can converse and eat detachedly at the same time. And you remember that it's not "you" tasting the food; it's the *taste buds* that taste the food, while it's the higher you, the conscious you, the powerful you, the slimmer you – that *witnesses* the taste buds tasting the food. Thus the "you" remains above and distinct from the food. Aloof from it. Above it all. You're one step removed from the food. No longer caught up or engrossed in food. The "you" no longer eats emotionally; you now eat consciously, impersonally – from reality, clarity, power, healthfulness and slimness. You're not just eating; you're intensely *aware* that you're eating. You know that you know you're eating.

And all while, that "witness" of yours, that sixth sense, that all-controlling master sense remains acutely aware, like a cat at a mouse-hole, for the very first inkling that the hunger has subsided – that the edge has been taken off, then you *stop eating immediately!* The body is finished eating.

The hand returns the fork to the plate for the last time, and you're delighted to notice that the body has become fully sated on a third of the food on that plate. How wonderful! The emotional attachment is broken. The mental obsession is lifted. The obstruction is removed. Deliverance has come.

Then you rest awhile in pleased satisfaction and gratitude – that you're now in control of food and that no longer does food control you. And with a big inner smile of pride and joy, you have the server package those leftovers to enjoy later. How sweet it is to be finally free. You feel good about your life now, and the pounds drop as planned, never to return.

Key Points and Principles:

1. That you were habituated from infancy to eat for emotional comfort and security.

2. That this wrong relationship with food causes overeating.

3. That overeating against your will is a condition in which your appetite is controlled subconsciously instead of consciously.

4. That this habit/behavior can be broken by witnessing every aspect of the eating experience from a *distance* instead of emotional attachment.

5. That thoughts and feelings are also controlled by keeping a conscious *distance* from them.

6. That "willpower" doesn't work on subconscious habits; only detached awareness works.

7. That you eat slowly and detachedly, while watching very

intently for the exact moment the hunger to subsides, then you stop eating immediately.

8. That "keeping your distance" is the universal key to self- and appetite-control.

9. That you never eat to fullness, but only to *take the edge off*.

10. That any distraction from the Method will cause you to overeat.

CHAPTER 2
PLANNING TO EAT, EATING TO PLAN

"You don't have to have a brain; you just have to know the road." – Scarecrow, *The Wizard of Oz*

The Plan Is The Thing

The last chapter spoke of *how* to eat to break the overeating habit, control your appetite and consequently lose weight. This chapter deals with the nuts and bolts, administrative and supportive part of your powerful, new, living and eating lifestyle. A plan gives order and structure to your day and removes much of the stress and personal discretion from the decision-making process.

Much of your day is already conducted by plan: Rising at a certain time and way; getting the children off to school, getting to work on time by a certain route, then working all day according to a plan prescribed by the job description, doing laundry and food shopping on certain days and times, etc. Daily food planning should be no less a natural, integral, routine part of your day – at least equal in importance to all other activities. And if you want to lose weight, then it should take an even higher priority than most all other activities. So let food planning be an integral part of your daily routine. Remember that "failing to plan is planning to fail." Get in the habit of doing everything "by the numbers" like the military does. It's a simpler, more intelligent and efficient way to live.

Losing Weight Incrementally

An effective strategy is to lose weight in five-to ten-pound increments instead of in a one, long, single span. Losing 50-pounds seems a daunting task, psychologically, but losing just five to ten pounds at a time seems more easily doable.

You can revert to "maintenance mode" for about a week in-between plateaus that you've reached. You'll find it easy to maintain your loss during them because your stomach has considerably shrunk. This will give added confidence and motivation as you move on to the next plateau.

Weight Loss Versus Weight Maintenance

In this Program, the difference between losing weight and maintaining the loss is simply one of *stringency*. When you stop overeating via the Method prescribed here, you'll stop gaining weight immediately. This is what we'll call "maintenance mode." This is how you should've been eating all along but didn't know how or didn't want to know. This program is actually a lifelong "maintenance mode" program.

To *lose* weight, however, you'll temporarily have to be a little more strict and rigorous in applying the Method. But that'll be much easier to do now because you've effectively "stopped the bleeding." *It's only when you've stopped overeating can you begin to start losing weight.*

For example, during the lifelong maintenance phase, you're qualified to "cheat" on occasion. By *cheating* I mean you can eat anything in moderation because now you're qualifed and capable of eating in moderation instead of overeating. You'll know how to control yourself and your appetite through several months experience and training in the Method.

So you can now be less exacting in your diet. You can have a slice of strawberyy cheesecake or blueberry muffin with your coffee, or overindulge at a wedding or on cruise with it's 24-hour buffett. You can have some cheese and crackers at "Happy Hour." You can have a slice of pizza or some baked lasagna with focaccia, or sample a French or Italian pastry for dessert, etc.

– But you can't eat *any* of these things during the weight loss phase because, again, you're not yet qualified by virtue of not having reached your goal weight yet nor having mastered appetite control via the Method yet. Once you know how to control yourself you can eat anything; but the wonderful thing is – you won't want to eat anything. You'll have lost your taste, interest and requirement for unhealthy, junk or "comfort" foods. Foods high in fat, sugar and carbs.

Eating Five Meals A Day

This Program prescribes eating *five times per day*. This means eating about every two and a half hours. For example, at about 8:00, 10:30, 1:00, 3:30 and 6:00 P.M. I have my clients choose and note down the five times they'll eat. Five meals daily keeps the fat-burning metabolism running on high and frees you from feeling deprived throughout the day.

Do remember that a "meal" in the context of this Program can mean a total of just three to six ounces of food. That may be – and usually is, all that's necessary to *take the edge off your hunge*r for that particular meal.

You should eat breakfast within one-hour of waking because your metabolism has slowed during the night, and breakfast will rev it up again. You should also have your last meal at least three-hours before bedtime so your food can fully digest before then. Going to sleep with a full stomach makes it easier for fat to establish a storage space – especially around the mid-section. Another caveat is that digestion uses lots of energy which may also interfere with the quality of your sleep. And a good night's sleep is integral to good health in general and waking refreshed and energized in particular.

Sample Menu Schedule (Weight-loss Phase)

Not clear on how to plan your menu? The guidline menu below is based on just three principles: Get protein with every meal, have at least two servings of fruit or veggies at each meal, and choose fiber-rich carbs. Unsweetened beverages like coffee, iced tea, and diet soft drinks are unlimited. (Careful, though, Aspartame has been proven to be an addictive substance.)

Average your calories out to about 1,600 per day, enough to help you lose weight slowly. Then, as you reach your goal weight, increase portion sizes of fruits, vegetables, and whole grains, and add a little more healthy fat to maintain that weight. Again, this is not a calorie-counting program but you do want to be *aware* of a particular meal's approximate calorie count.

My clients choose their own five, balanced, nutritious meals based on their own tastes, restrictions and research. Here's a sample guideline menu just to give you an idea:

(1) 8:00 A.M. (Breakfast):
    3 ounces protein
    1 starch/grain serving
    1 fruit serving
    1 cup dairy

(2) 10:30 A.M. (Mid-Morning Snack):
    2 ounces protein
    1 fruit serving
    1 cup dairy

(3) 1:00 P.M. (Lunch):
    3 ounces protein
    1 starch/grain serving
    1 fruit serving
    3 vegetable servings
    2 fat servings

(4) 3:30 P.M. (Mid-Afternoon Snack):
    2 ounces protein
    1 fruit serving
    1 cup dairy

(5) 6:00 P.M. (Dinner):
    3 ounces protein,
    1 starch/grain serving
    1 fruit serving,
    3 vegetable servings
    2 fat servings

Don't Even Think About Eating Between Meals

The Program prescribes *no eating between meals* – not even an olive! Here's why: When you eat something, even something as innocent as a celery stalk, for example, it signals the salivary glands, stomach and small intestine to start releasing about twenty-two enzymes and acids to help with the digestion and absorption process. All systems are go, and they anticipate and *expect* more food to come down the pike. No more food is coming but they wait and wait and wait; and this waiting, this expectation, is felt as a craving for food. But the body isn't necessarily hungry! You simply tempted and excited the digestive system with that innocent celery stalk!

Overcoming Cravings

You may be one of those people who have mistakenly believed that between-meal eating urges occur because of physical withdrawal and because you *need* to eat. But that isn't true. Most of our urges or hunger pangs are triggered by unrelated things, like the time of day, certain people we're around, a type of feeling, or the kids coming home. Cravings or urges are simply conditioned responses that seldom last very long. And when you don't indulge them they get weaker and weaker and easier to ignore. So when you feel a craving or apparent hunger pang, you can talk to yourself in your mind, reminding yourself that in a minute or two it'll pass. And it always does.

Your subconscious mind will remind you that you don't ever have to indulge any urges, and almost before you realize it, the cravings are gone. And that's going to be a delight, discovering that eating urges and hunger pangs quickly pass, and you don't have to robotically react to them as you have in the past.

You Can Always Tell An Overeater, But You Can't Tell Him Much!

Most people don't like to be told what they can or can't do or eat – even when we're telling it to ourselves, we don't like it. It's human nature to rebel against restrictions of any kind. But instead of struggling with a between-meal craving, you can just watch it from a little distance, and in a few minutes it'll pass. They're just a signal to let you know that you need to cope with this situation. And you cope with it by detachedly watching it instead of fighting it.

The only thing that makes it difficult is your telling yourself that it is. But as you reaffirm your commitment to respect and protect your body, you'll find cravings occur less and are less uncomfortable. And you can remind yourself that if you don't eat that chocolate cake at that particular moment, you're not going to disintegrate. You can handle it. Anybody can. So what if it's not pleasant or easy sometimes? Life itself is not always pleasant and easy. You can handle a little brief discomfort from time to time – easpecially when it's for such a worthy cause – your health, happiness, self-esteem and slimmer body. Every worthwhile goal in life has a price and this is a very small price to pay to achieve your goal. It's a terrific bargain. And you feel so good about yourself afterwards, don't you?

Breathing Away Your Cravings

If for any reason you feel the desire to eat between your five regular meals, just stop, close your eyes and take three deep breaths, and that feeling will dissolve and disappear. This works because your breathing is directly related to your central nervous system, and when your nerves are relaxed, your so-called cravings are relaxed as well.

Your indifference to cravings puts them behind you. You ignore them, reject them, deny them. You refuse to claim them. Refuse to accept them as real. Refuse to buy them. Refuse to fall for them. You don't reckon with them whatsoever. You don't entertain them or believe them for a second. You don't fight them, resist them or recognize them. Just take three deep breaths and immediately let them go, let them disappear into the nothingness that they really are. And you do this calmly, naturally and with total conviction.

A Craving Faced Is A Craving Erased

Experience any between-meal craving fully and indifferently. When an urge arises to eat between meals, again, don't be averse to it, but enter into it with relish. Make it a meditation. Look it straight in the eye with firm, poised dispassion and watch it dissolve. "A pain faced is a pain erased." Catch the urge at the point of inception. Notice what you're doing at the time – what the trigger is – then stop doing it. Just freeze on the spot and detachedly observe it. Be a witness to it as if it were not happening to *you* but just happening, period.

See it as something that's not really you, not really real. Just because you feel it doesn't make it real. *The feeling is real but it's falsely based because you're body isn't really hungry.* See the difference? The feeling came from your imagination or your past conditioning – not from reality!

Passively watch the so-called craving as if watching a movie on a screen, then click the pause button to freeze-frame it. Just witness it without the slightest desire that it leave. Don't entertain or indulge it as real. No longer exert effort or willpower. No longer empower it by fighting or resisting it. At that point the craving leaves you. It vaporizes into the nothingness it really is.

By experiencing a discomfort to the end you are disproving its reality and its power. Passive, detached energy works like a light that makes the dark disappear. As darkness is merely the absence of light so pain is merely the absence of detached mindfulness. By shining indifferent attention on a craving, its nothingness, its un-substantialness becomes exposed. Then, just take three deep breaths and go back about your business.

Drinking Six To Eight Glasses of Water Per Day

Drinking pure, clear, uncolored water many times per day will free your body from the need to retain fluids. It'll wash away fatty toxins and cellulite. It will make you feel more refreshed and energized, and will diminish between-meal cravings. Many cravings for food are actually a thirst for water!

Portion Controlling

Formal "weighing and measuring" is not required during the *Maintenance Phase* of this Program because the method itself *is* the portion controller! During the weight-losing phase, however, there are three factors you'll need to take into consideration – which are based on the human condition that "the spirit is willing but the flesh is weak."

One is that your thoughts, feelings and eyes will *always* be larger than your stomach – which is only about the size of a closed fist; two, that the problem for the beginner is overcoming the *temptation* to keep on eating after satiety has been reached. Orson Welles said, "I can resist anything except temptation." And three, there's the build-up of *momentum* while eating that has to be checked. – A mouth in motion tends to stay in motion.

For these reasons, portion-controlling is required during the weight-*losing* phase of the Program. The idea is this: If there's nothing on your plate, it's difficult to eat it. Again, once you've reached goal weight, it won't matter how much food is on your plate – measured or not, because you'll be established and experienced enough in the *Three-Phase Method* to stop at the correct moment.

Another important caveat is that your hunger may be sated *before* you've finished your "measured" portion, so stopping eating via the Method would always take precedence over stopping via portion control. Just because it's the "correct" portion doesn't mean you have to eat it. Portion control is just a guideline or reference – not a license or loophole to continue eating.

Calorie Counting

You won't need to count calories either, for the same reason, but do be *aware* of the amount of calories, fat and sugars in a given meal or snack. Remember that this is an *awareness* program not a diet program. Diets don't work; awareness – *detached* awareness, always does. And as this is a lifelong program, keeping it simple is key to success.

As you're likely to always have leftovers, it's a good idea to keep a few food containers handy. Keeping them right on the table next to your dinner plate is good strategy. The idea, again, is to take all personal discretion out of the eating experience.

Remember that your eating behavior is driven by your subconscious program, not the logical, rational, intelligent part of your mind. So, again, the amount of food you "think" or "feel" you need will *always* be excessive; therefore, you can't ever trust those faculties in this matter.

Even though you're replacing a bad habit with a good one, it'll still feel awkward in the beginning, as all new habits do. Be patient. Psychologists say it takes about twenty-one days for a new habit to become assimilated. But assimilation happens much faster and deeper in this Program because we'll be using powerful self-hypnosis, guided meditation and visualization techniques to greatly enhance and facilitate the process.

Advance Meal Planning

Another essential part of the Program is to *plan all your meals in advance.* You have a choice of two methods – plan five meals in advance for the day, or 28 meals in advance for the week. Many of my clients say the "one day at a time" approach is the most simple and effective because it aligns with the body's natural biorhythm, and because life does happen one day at a time. Build a thick, brick wall around your day and eat and live within it. It makes shopping easier, too. It eliminates the disorder and risk of having to make choices on whim or while hungry. You could plan the night before or first thing in the morning.

The efficacy of advance meal planning is the same as for

portion control. It removes mental and emotional (personal) considerations from the food-choosing and eating process. You eat according to nutritional needs rather than mood or caprice. There's nothing to think about; you just follow the instructions. Remember the five P's: "Prior Planning Prevents Poor Performance."

Making a Hit List

It's also helpful to make a list of those foods that you know are not healthy and avoid them, especially those foods and ingredients you know are your "trigger" or "binge" foods – those foods that you eat in large quantities or to the exclusion of other foods; foods that you turn to in times of celebration, sadness, stress or boredom; or foods that are high in calories and low in nutritional value. In addition, look to see whether there are any common ingredients among those foods – like refined sugar or fat that might exist in foods you haven't listed.

Below are examples of foods and eating behaviors that have been known to cause excessive cravings. Each of us may have problems with different foods or ingredients. If a food has been a binge food in the past, or if it contains ingredients that have been binge foods for you, remove it from your plan. For example, if pasta is a trigger food, then other foods made with flour (breads, muffins, crackers) could cause problems. Extra servings of a non-trigger food might create cravings. If you are unsure whether a food causes problems for you, leave it out at first.

Here are some examples: "Comfort" foods or junk foods such as chocolate, name-brand fast foods, cookies, potato chips. Foods containing refined sugar such as desserts, sweetened drink products and cereals, many processed meats, many condiments. Foods containing fats such as butter, cheese and other high-fat dairy or non-dairy foods, deep-fried foods and snacks, and many desserts. Foods containing wheat or flour or refined carbs in general such as pastries, certain pastas and breads. Foods containing mixtures of sugar and fat, or sugar, flour and fat such as ice cream, doughnuts, cakes and pies. Foods you eat in large quantities even though they aren't your trigger foods.

When you identify the foods and ingredients that cause you cravings, you simply stop eating them. Remember that you are the boss of your body. As you practice patience, perseverance – and *detached awareness*, your interest in wrong foods and behaviors will leave you without effort or willpower. Remember also that *nothing tastes as good as being thinner feels*.

Keeping a Journal

Another essential part of the Program is to *keep a daily record* of what you eat and drink. This gives you perspective, objectivity and accountability. It helps you take a clear and critical look at your food habits when the concentrated action of eating is over. Writing down what you just ate allows you to deal with food in a relaxed, organized way. Your journal will help you to recognize why and when you eat the foods you do. And it'll provide the means to discern the nutrient content and balance of your food.

Each day, note everything you ate at every meal – as soon as possible after the meal. You don't want to rely on memory because it's too convenient to "forget" eating the wrong food or amount at the wrong time. Be specific. And most important – be honest! Nothing is more slimming than honesty and integrity. It's the spiritual flavor that makes everything fall into place for you.

Relapsing Is Part of The Program

Slips will happen. When they do, simply note them down and think *nothing* of it. Never berate yourself. Never doubt yourself. Never feel guilt or shame about any food-related experience. These emotions are a contradiction of the principle that, subconsciously, you're *already* at your goal weight, and will sabotage the "creative" process.

"Slips" will occur less and less frequently. Notice how time, place, situation and certain people you're with affect what and how much you ate. For instance, were you driving, at a business luncheon, at a restaurant, on a cruise, alone or with others? Remember that any distraction will result in your overeating because the mind can't be in two places at the same time. If you eat while watching TV, for example, it's guaranteed you'll overeat no matter how great a multi-tasker you "think" you are. This is because overeating is the "norm" for you. It's your unconscious, default eating behavior. The whole purpose of the Method is simply to make you more conscious of your eating – detachedly conscious. It's really as simple as that.

Notice your mood – angry, bored, tired, lonely, stressed, rushed, excited, etc. Notice, especially, that you tend to eat less and better food simply by virtue of recording it. Your journal becomes an angelic friend – warding off temptation and gently nudging you on the straight and narrow path toward good health, good appearance, joy and freedom.

Weighing Yourself Daily

Weigh yourself every day at the same time and record it in your journal. Your scale and journal are the most powerful allies your beautiful new way of life could have. Your scale doesn't lie or make excuses. Remember that it's normal for your weight to fluctuate one to four pounds per day.

The Limitation-Is-Freedom Principle

All this planning won't be as burdensome or stifling as it may seem. In fact, it'll be quite the opposite. It'll be more liberating because you won't have to think about food all the time, obsess about it any longer. Your eating life will be settled in advance, so you can forget about it and go on with other areas of your life. This will free you up to get a life – a life beyond food. These controls add rhyme, reason and order to your eating life. It frees you by limiting you. *You just eat slowly and detachedly, watching very attentively for the exact point the edge has been taken off – then immediately stop and wrap the leftovers!*

Rewarding Yourself

Your mind-body transformation will be its own reward, but till you get there, rewarding yourself along the way with a little pat on the back is highly motivating. Mary Kay Ash said, "There are two things people want more than sex or money – recognition and praise!" And recognition begins at home, so for each increment or short-term goal that's achieved, have a planned reward set up in advance. Here are a few suggestions: Enjoy a day at the spa with a hot-rock massage and sauna; enjoy dinner at a fine French restaurant; buy a new (smaller) suit, dress or exercise outfit; treat yourself to a night on the town; get a pedicure; go to a play or concert; buy a smoothie machine or a new cookbook; relax and enjoy a candle-lit bubble bath with a bottle of Champagne, etc.

Key Points and Principles:

1. The purpose of a plan is to remove (detach) personal discretion from the decision-making /eating process.

2. Pre-plan all meals, daily or weekly.

3. Weigh/measure all meals to prevent temptation and momentum (during the weight-loss phase).

4. When determining when to stop eating, the *Method* takes precedence over any "measured" portion.

5. Be *aware* of a food's fat, sugar and calorie content but counting is optional.

6. During the weight loss phase: Eat by the Method 5 times daily with nothing in between.

7. Drink 6-8 glasses of water per day.

8. List and avoid known binge or trigger foods.

9. Record/journal all meals to maintain awareness, objectivity and accountability.

10. Weigh yourself daily at the same time.

11. Think absolutely nothing of occasional slips.

12. Reward your patient progress regularly.
13. Plan to lose weight in 5- to 10-pound increments.

CHAPTER 3
REVISING YOUR SELF-IMAGE

*"Self-image sets the boundaries of
individual accomplishment."* – Maxwell Maltz, MD

Perception Is Reality

Overeating, like any other habit, good or bad, is "programmed" into the subconscious memory-bank part of your mind. This subconscious program runs your eating behavior automatically just as other programs run your respiratory, digestive, healing and immune systems, etc., automatically.

Your overeating habit can be stopped at will, simply by "saying the word," just by telling your subconscious mind to stop it. After all, you are the boss of your body – but you have to communicate it in a way that the subconscious mind can understand.

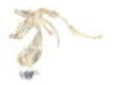

How the Subconscious Mind Works

The first thing to understand about the subconscious is that it doesn't have a mind of it's own, so to speak. It doesn't judge, analyze or use logic as your conscious mind does. It only knows what you tell it, and whatever you tell it is accepted as absolute truth. – Which is why we have to be careful and conscious of what we tell it. It can easily misinterpret things. For example, if you were taking a short-cut home through your neighbor's strawberry patch, and you bent over to tie your shoes – that would give the impression, perception or image to anyone watching, that you were stealing strawberries, wouldn't it? And if you claimed you were just tying your shoes, no one would believe you. For the subconscious mind, the *image* of stealing is the *same* as actually stealing. It has the same effect. So for the subconscious mind, image *is* reality. Perception *is* everything.

Here's another example: You're walking along a country road, and a large twig falls from a tree just in front of you, and you "think" it's a snake! You become very frightened. Petrified. Your heart rate soars, your adrenalin starts pumping, you break out into a cold sweat – but it's only a twig! This is how the imagination alone can effect and control the body. And this is how, if you can *convince* your subconscious that you weigh 150 pounds when you really weigh 200 pounds, it will work around the clock, knocking down all the blockages, to get you to 150 pounds!

Getting What You Give

In other words, the subconscious mind sees and functions just like a computer program or mirror: If you give it "I can't do this," it will reflect in your behavior "You can't do this"; If you give it "food makes me feel better," it will give you "food makes you feel better"; if you give it, "I am fat," it will give you and keep you fat.

Whatever negative thing you think, feel or say about

yourself will become or remain the truth of your experience. Virtually all the negativity and limitation in your life is unconsciously self-created. What you "believe" creates a self-fulfilling prophecy. Here's a brief sampling of common false beliefs and self-imposed limitations that will sabotage your weight loss and general self-improvement efforts every time:

- I have a hormonal imbalance!
- I don't have the patience!
- I don't deserve it!
- This is my default weight!
- It's hereditary!
- No matter what I do...!
- I just can't stop eating!
- Sweets are my weakness!
- I have a fear of failure!
- I have a fear of success!
- I'm just an overweight type of person!
- I always gain the weight back!
- I don't have the self-confidence!
- I'm a "glass is half-empty" type of person!
- I can't get organized!
- If I get my hopes up, I'll just be disappointed!
- I'm not self-motivated!
- I'm a procrastinator!
- I should be further along by now!
- I hate to exercise!
- I'm an addictive type personality!
- I have a weakness for...!
- I'm stuck on this plateau!

- I'm a compulsive overeater!
- I'm big-boned!

Every item on this list, in fact, every negative thing you've ever thought about yourself – is absolutely not true! *It's all in your mind*. All self-manufactured. All in the six or seven inches between your left ear and your right ear. In reality there's nothing, absolutely nothing in the universe that is negative. All negativity of any name or nature is *self-created*. So if you think or feel that you're anything on this list, then stop thinking or feeling that way. Just stop it. There's no how. Just stop it!

The essential point is this: If you look in the mirror and think or feel that there's something wrong about yourself or your body, or that you are overweight, then *you're going to stay overweight for as long as you think that!* So if you want to change how you look, feel and eat, you'll have to change your "self-image" accordingly. You'll have to imagine yourself *already* looking, feeling, eating and weighing what you want. Your body follows your image like the caboose follows the engine. This is what's meant by, "It's all in your mind." It's because the subconscious mind is totally controlled by you, just as you are totally controlled by it. They mirror-reflect each other. So if you want to know how to conduct yourself, conduct yourself according this all-powerful, universal law.

Self-image Is Your Mind-Body Creator

Your self-image is what's feeding and maintaining that body, so a new and improved self-image is how you're going to begin to change it. Your body will emulate your thinking whether that thinking is right or wrong, true or false. So if you're striving for a goal that contradicts what you "think" you presently are, then your subconscious must and will figure out a way to obstruct or sabotage your efforts. Your subconscious mirror reflects that you're overweight because that's what you put in front of it. Using the computer metaphor, your subconscious computer calculates that being overweight is what you want because that's the information you unwittingly gave it, so it'll work to make you *gain* more weight. This explains why we tend to overeat at the same time we've decided to lose weight.

This is a common phenomenon in sports improvement where, for example, you're a golfer with a self-image handicap of a certain number. This is *your* number, *your* handicap. Then one day, when not thinking much about your game, you greatly improve on it. Then you smile and think, no, no. This is not like me. Not the real me. Not my handicap. Just some kind of fluke. So you then, *unconsciously*, proceed to hit a few balls into water and sand traps in order bring your handicap back to where it was before. Where it coincides with your pre-determined "self-image" handicap and comfort zone.

Convincing The Subconscious Mind

You change your self-image by *convincing* the subconscious mind that you're *not* overweight. It will then slap immediate controls on your appetite to make this imaginary fact real.

In changing your self-image, there are several elements to understand and follow. The first element is to mentally change from your present weight to your desired weight – which we'll refer to as your "default" weight. You want to see and feel yourself as your ideal weight right *here-now*, even though your "logical" mind tells you that you're really not.

This is because what your logical mind "thinks" doesn't matter. *Your logical mind didn't get you overweight and won't get you thinner* – as you may have noticed. You can't use the same mind that caused the problem to correct it. That's why you have to use your subconscious imagination instead of logic. Logic is doing what you've always done – like dieting, because that's how you've always done it. Your vivid imagination has the power to override or transcend logic to bring your goal to realization. So it's not about changing your diet program; it's about changing your subconscious-mind program.

Relaxing Your Guard

The way to neutralize that entrenched, eating-for-comfort security guard is simply to *relax* her. Relax her to the point her guard is down enough to allow your new weight to be accepted into your creative subconscious mind. That's the germination point where the blooming of the new you can begin.

The way to access the subconscious part of your mind is by relaxing the conscious part. The conscious part is almost always moving – constantly thinking, reasoning, desiring, analyzing, rationalizing, conceptualizing – while the subconscious part is constantly *still*. The idea is to still the conscious mind to the same level as is the subconscious mind. That's the point of exchange when your goal affirmation can transfer to it. The process is like that of an airplane being refueled in midair by another airplane. The transfer of fuel can only take place when both planes are moving at the same speed at the same time. Or think of the opening of the subconscious mind as the eye of a relaxed sewing needle, and the conscious mind as a nervous length of thread. The thread must be stilled before it can pass through the eye of the needle.

Communicating With Your Source of Power

The relationship between the conscious and subconscious minds is a communication process much like that between a radio receiver and transmitter. The transmitter is like the subconscious. It is the *source* of all intelligence and goal-achievement power. And the receiver is like the conscious mind. Its job is to be *receptive* to the source. It can't be receptive, however, unless it's tuned into the transmitter, and it can't unless it's still or relaxed.

When we're excited or stressed, it's as if we're chaotically and indiscriminately moving the dial hither and dither without ever coming to rest, and so receiving only gibberish as a result. We're scattered rather than focused.

Or think of the conscious and subconscious minds as the two sections of an hourglass: The subconscious is the top half, and only about seven-percent at a time can ever flow into consciousness, the bottom half. The narrow-minded (biased) neck restricts the flow. As we become more open-minded via detachment, we in effect, widen the neck of the hourglass until it becomes like a water glass. Now, what's above is the same as below. Now there's no difference between the top-half and the bottom-half. Now they are one whole, not two halves. One mind, not two minds. There's no separation, obstruction, conflict or distinction between them. What was subconscious now becomes conscious.

At that point, you are empowered! Whatever state of body or mind you want is yours, first imaginatively, then in due course, physically. You realize natural and effortless appetite-control power, and the excess weight drops of its own accord. Or in the case of other eating disorders, the behavior falls away on its own. It just gives up on you because you're no longer feeding or empowering it.

The "Happiness-First" Principle

We can now move on to the next element in the mind/body transformation process. Earlier I defined an "eating disorder" as the condition when the mind follows the body instead of vice versa. This means that you have to change your mind before the body can change. So we're not talking at all about "dieting" here – that's putting the body first instead of the mind first, which is the erroneous, upside-down approach guaranteed to fail every time. The correct approach is to begin at the *end* not the beginning. By the "end" we not only mean your goal weight, we also and especially mean *the state of mind to which your goal will bring you* – and that's a state of *happiness.*

Yes, achieving your goal will make you happy, but the catch – the paradoxical law governing the creative process is that *you must be happy before you can control your appetite and lose that weight.* Happiness is the seed; weight loss is the fruit. You have to be happy in the first place before you can lose weight in the second place.

So what's the definition of happiness in this context? Happiness is a condition of *perfect contentment and peace of mind* in which there are no needs or desires – including the desire to lose weight. It means that right now you are whole and complete. Nothing is lacking or missing in you.

You want to cultivate an attitude of *unconditional happiness* in which nothing can upset or disturb you. One thing doesn't affect you any more than another. "Keeping your distance" from all that you see, hear, think, feel and do, is the natural way to achieve and maintain this state of mind. If you find it difficult to be unconditionally happy all the time, then practice the old adage to "fake it till you make it." *Act* unconditionally happy until you really are. This "acting is if" is another technique for changing your subconscious mind. Your subconscious will eventually incorporate the idea. Again, if you're sad about achieving your goal, your subconscious will think you're sad about losing weight and will try to help you gain it back. So don't be sad about anything. Keep your life on an even keel by remaining above it all. This is the enlightened and empowering attitude of happiness, joy, freedom and a slimmer body.

How to Desire

The paradoxical problem in achieving your goal is that emotional desire is almost always accompanied with stress or anxiety. They come as a package – two sides of the same coin. Desire contradicts contentment. Desire indicates something's missing. There's a lack or deficiency. Whenever you feel in want or need of something, you leave the realm of relaxed and joyful contentedness and become tense like a tightly stretched rubber band. You become off-center, unbalanced, and you remain so until that goal is fulfilled, satisfied or resolved in some way. The *emotional* effort to achieve that goal is what strengthens the disorder's grip on you. It's exactly what hinders success.

We are almost always stressed because we are almost always wanting something or other. The human being is a virtual *desiring machine*. We want to grow, improve, evolve, expand. We want more money, more security, more sex, more time, more space, more power. We want to improve our bridge game, have a better car, a better job, a better relationship, a bigger house, a faster computer. We want to get married or divorced, buy a boat or get rid of a boat, get justice or revenge, pass that test, improve our health, heal a disease, make a good impression, be right, be first, be famous, be more attractive, wiser and wittier; be more recognized, validated, admired, appreciated. We want to win the race, win the argument, get that promotion, retire early. The list is virtually endless and constant.

The conundrum is this: You're stressed *because* you emotionally want something, and that clarity-blocking stress is exactly what prevents you from getting it. It's a vicious cycle. So the essential question becomes – how can you *desire* to lose weight without the failure-causing stress that comes with it? In other words, how can you be happy *before* you lose that weight, so that you *can* lose that weight?

The Principle of "Already-Being-There"

The answer lies in knowing *the right way to desire*. It's about knowing the law- or reality-based way to ask yourself for the weight or eating behavior that you want. Your computer-like subconscious requires certain criteria be met before it can process your order. The first is that you order with the right attitude, and the right attitude is to assume, believe and accept that you *already* have, right now, whatever you desire to be, do or have in the future. Again, you have to be there in mind before you can be there in body – as discussed earlier. You have to mentally and emotionally accept as a foregone conclusion, as a *fait accompli*, that your goal has *already* been achieved, that it's a done deal, that it's finished.

This attitude of "already-being-there" transcends the desire-stress-failure vicious cycle. You are now like a plane flying above the storm. You're now, in effect, not only happily content in the *process* of losing that weight, you're now most effective in losing it. Emotional-control *is* appetite-control. They are one and the same state of mind. You're unstoppable because you're living above and detached from all that could or would block you. Assuming that you've "already arrived" empowers your subconscious to make it happen in actuality by removing failure-causing emotionality from the goal-achievement process.

You are formulating your desire in a way that conforms with how the imaginative, creative faculty is designed to work, with how the subconscious mind is actually wired. You are in compliance with subconscious law.

The Subconscious Is Wired To Fulfill Your Desire

Now everything in the universe works according to law and order, and the mind is no exception. The law of your mind, that is, your higher, subconscious mind, is that it *must* give you whatever you want or need. You are the law of yourself, the boss of yourself, the boss of your body. Think of the subconscious as your personal computer and you are its master programmer. Whatever you say, goes. You just have to say it in the right way – beginning with the attitude you *already* have it.

Here's a variation of an old Zen story that illustrates the above point: An American woman, despairingly overweight for many years, traveled to the Himalayas to seek the counsel of a famous wise woman. After much searching, she found her walking up a steep hill. The American struggled to catch up to her.

The wise woman said, "Why do you want to see me?"

The American said, "Please, I want to lose weight. I want to lose weight."

"The way to lose weight," said the wise woman, "can be stated in five words."

"Five words? But, I've traveled such a long way," said the American. "Can you give me more than just five words?"

"I can give you ten-thousand words if you like, but they would boil down to the same five words."

"Okay," said the American. "I've tried everything. Tell me what to do and I'll do it. What are the five words?"

"Just drop the '*I want*,'" said the wise woman.

You overcome the vicious circle by getting out of the way of it. You put your lower, personal, emotional self aside, in order to fulfill the law and achieve your goal. You have to separate yourself from what you want in order for your higher, subconscious self, to proceed to give it to you. *"Keeping your distance"* again and again, is the master key to the emotional-control that *is* appetite-control, that *is* living in reality. It's removing yourself from, or rising above, the emotional desire to lose that weight by assuming and accepting that you've already lost it.

The Outcome Is None of Your Emotional Business

You're coming from success not from hunger or deficiency. Deficient is not who you are. That's a deception. You are whole and complete, just as the universe is. So all your desires and goals are merely recreational activities that can't fail to be achieved because on some level, they already are. That's the reality-based way to think of them.

You are now, in effect, emotionally uninvolved regarding the end result. It's not a factor in the success equation. You are totally indifferent and dispassionate with respect to the whether or not you lose that weight. This is how you facilitate the achievement process rather than short-circuit or sabotage it. Henry James put it this way – "When once a decision is reached and execution is the order of the day, dismiss absolutely all responsibility and care about the outcome."

This principle has been taught by so many teachers so many times and in so many ways, from antiquity to the present, that is has become almost cliché. But don't get tired of hearing it for understanding and practicing it is the master key to losing all the weight that you want lose almost effortlessly.

Extricating yourself emotionally from your goal is the means by which to access the joy, clarity and creative power necessary to achieve that goal. The inspiration of the painter, poet, composer, entrepreneur, etc., comes only when she's able to view her work with emotional detachment. She becomes tense when ideas don't flow, and when they do, excitement prevents their sustainment. She suffers frustration because what she clearly knows in her mind and feels in her heart won't translate faithfully onto canvas or into words or music. She's blocked. Uncontrolled emotion has stifled her power of perception and expression.

The creative genius in any medium is one who has learned to overcome a restless mind and an anxious heart. She can maintain a serene indifference during both the creative feasts and famines alike; consequently, the famines occur less and less, and the feasts, more and more. The same principle of creative success applies to the appetite-control artist. Non-emotional involvement with food is the master key to gaining control over it.

The Cause of Failure

So-called failure is nothing but positive feedback, to inform you that you've gone astray. It's the result of consciously or unconsciously breaking some universal law. It's the penalty you pay for either disobedience or ignorance of the law. If you're not losing weight as intended or not maintaining your weight loss, it's because you're not in compliance with *the law of detachment*. There's no other reason because the law itself is absolutely infallible. It's simply not possible to overeat and be detachedly aware at the same time. They're contradictory activities. It's like when you turn the light on, the darkness has to turn off.

Just let the subconscious do all the work. Keep your lower, personal self out of the picture. Your best thinking got you into this situation; don't depend on it to get you out of it. Only when you are above and separate from your feelings can your feelings be controlled and your desire granted. It's granted first on the subconscious level the moment you ask in this way, then, in due course, it's granted in actuality – on the physical level. In other words, you control your emotions in order to control the outcome, and you control your emotions by keeping a *distance* from them.

To assume you're "already there" entails *visualizing what you'll look and feel like at your goal weight*. Creative imagination is the forming of a picture in the mind's eye of what you want to be, do or have. In cinematic terms, you'd be creating a "trailer" of your future body, or a "preview of coming attractions." Or we could say, "A preview of coming attractiveness." Imagining a thing is prerequisite to having it in actuality. This is creative law, and it applies to creating the mind and body that you really want, just as to creating the vacation, house, business and relationships that you really want.

Right and Wrong Motivation

Let's clarify a few foundational points before you begin to visualize your present-future body. First, the creative process requires that you desire to achieve your goal for the right reason or right motivation. The right motivation gives you the necessary resoluteness and firmness of purpose to overwrite the long-established false program that keeps you in the grip of your eating disorder.

Ineffective reasons to lose weight would be, for example, to fit into that great suit you bought on sale, or to look better at your daughter's wedding, or for that Caribbean cruise, etc.

A less obvious wrong reason for losing weight would be for

your health. That's right. Health is not a good enough reason for your subconscious mind because your subconscious is not about effects; it's about *causes*. It's not about fear of heart disease or diabetes; it's about being who you really are at the center of your being. Who you really are is *not* overweight, is not the *real* you, is not the truth of your being.

And that's the primary criterion necessary to activate and energize your subconscious power. Everything else is just wishful thinking and useless rationalizing. The whole will and purpose of the subconscious mind is to facilitate your being your real and higher self – which is *not* overweight. You just have to learn how to get out of the way and let it happen. *"Keeping your distance"* from all you think, feel, do and eat, is how you get out of the way.

Right and Wrong Conviction

Think of your subconscious mind as the negative film in a camera. In order to impress upon it the *picture* of the mind and body you want, the light of your desire has to be sufficiently intense.

Controlling your appetite has to be your heart's burning, dominant desire. It can't be a casual or superficial whim. You have to be irrevocably and unwaveringly determined as well as happily detached and centered. Gaining control of your mind and body has to be the number-one priority in your life, not only for itself, but also because it affects every other area of your life. Along with your appearance and health, it affects your self-confidence, self-esteem and self-image. It affects your relationships, your finances, your work and your play.

And this determination, when practiced correctly, is not at all stressful or willful. It's perfectly smooth and natural. It means you're now focused instead of scattered. Remember that the right conviction and mindset is that your goal is *already* achieved. That's what you have to make up your mind to. Stress enters the equation only when a goal has not yet been achieved – when the desired result is a future unknown. Know also that this is not some kind of mental gimmick, but is the way the subconscious mind and *the law of detachment* work. It's the way we were designed for optimal functioning.

Right and Wrong Use of Willpower

Many people on the path of recovery from their food issues cite a lack of sufficient willpower as the main reason for their setbacks. But they have plenty of willpower or they wouldn't have tried so many remedies so many times. The problem is they just don't know how to use it. The incorrect understanding and use of willpower is the most common reason for failure in any long-term endeavor

You may have noticed that whenever you've tried "willpower" to lose weight, you burned out quickly. You became drained, began to lose confidence and doubt yourself. Each time you attempt willpower to control yourself, you fail, and you fail sooner each time because you just know that you're going to fail – and of course, you will because you're using the wrong tool in the wrong way.

The two key points to understand about willpower are one, that willpower isn't designed for long-term use – such as running a marathon. It's designed only for short bursts of energy and adrenalin – like being able to lift a two-thousand pound car to save a child's life, for instance – but you wouldn't be able to hold that car up for very long, would you? And two, that willpower can only treat *symptoms* not causes. It's useful only on the physical and mental levels *not* on the subconscious level – where the habit is rooted.

The correct use of willpower is to practice the method of eating in a slow and detached way, watching attentively for the exact point the hunger has subsided, then stopping immediately! This is the only activity you have to master via personal willpower. Everything else in this book is peripheral and supportive of this one primary goal. If you learn only one thing in this book, learn this and you'll lose weight and keep it off forever.

Right and Wrong Attitudes

Your all-powerful, all-positive, subconscious mind is working full-time toward your goal, but its law or nature can be subverted by any kind of sustained negative thinking or feeling. These negativities will sabotage your plan, will contradict the law and make it impotent.

The two most egregious deal killers are *impatience and doubt.* Impatience is not living in reality because any kind of healing or change on the physical level must take time. Our lower human nature wants instant results. We want what we want, when we want it. And, of course, the stress of impatience causes you to eat even more, doesn't it?

And doubt means fear or lack of faith. Fear that you won't achieve your goal – mostly because of past failures. And faithlessness for the same reason. The obvious answer is to stop living in the past – which we'll discuss later.

Countless volumes have been written on the power of faith, and all of the greatest teachers of self-mastery throughout history have proved and taught the efficacy of faith. No matter how clear and strong your desire to lose that weight, if you don't *believe* that you can and will do it, then you can't and won't. It's simple mathematics. It's not only a state of mind; it's also a *choice* of mind. You can choose to believe you'll lose weight, or not. You want to doubt your doubts more and believe your beliefs more. If you don't have it yet, just *pretend* that you do until you really do. "Fake it till you make it," is the reality-based admonition to apply in this case.

Being Open-minded

Instead of doubting success, just be open to it. Amenable to it. Self-control is not something you do; it's something you *allow*. When you doubt or fear, you're effectively separating yourself from your goal. You are putting your ideal body on an emotional pedestal, programming yourself to remain always apart from it. Doubt puts your goal over the horizon somewhere where it must always remain. When you doubt, you're are like *Waiting for Godot*. Godot will never come. Waiting, trying and doubting then become a way of life, just as running from diet to diet becomes a way of life.

Doubting makes your goal an unattainable object, an ongoing exercise in futility and fantasy like a carrot held in front of one's nose. Either control your appetite or don't control it, but don't doubt and don't try. Just do it! The subconscious only understands do or die. It's a binary thing. Yes or no. Have or have not. It can't compute the indecisiveness, uncertainty and weakness of doubt, fear, hope, try or maybe. So doubt all your doubts and believe all your positive beliefs.

To be open-minded and acceptant is to be empty and receptive. Whenever you're empty, all that's necessary to achieve your goal will effortlessly rush in to fill the void. Emerson said, "Once you make a decision, the universe conspires to make it happen." If you want something, you have to make a space for it. That's what detachment does.

Your Subconscious Genie

The subconscious computer doesn't care or lean one way or the other. It's a totally indifferent, impersonal, free-will faculty. Whatever you tell it, it accepts. Whatever you ask of it in the right way, it *must* give you because that's its job, its primary purpose. Any fear, doubt or uncertainty about attaining this goal is asking incorrectly. It's asking with attachment to the goal. It's asking in a contradictory way – as if you don't already have it, and that's exactly what will prevent success. What else can be expected? The process has been sabotaged at its very inception. Disappointment is a forgone conclusion. Doubt, worry or uncertainty is virtually planning to fail, and so you will.

The subconscious mind will accept your goal mind and body exactly as presented, exactly as imagined, whether it's right or wrong, true or false, healthy or unhealthy. It isn't at all logical like the conscious mind. It doesn't discriminate, analyze, rationalize or judge. If you ask for something in the right way – the detached, desireless way prescribed here, it will be granted. Period. It is the law of cause and effect.

So faith is really more scientific than commonly

understood. It's just as exact a science as mathematics. Just because you can't see the future doesn't mean it doesn't exist. And not only does it exist, but you can create it or re-create it the way you want it. If you can imagine it, you can have it. And nothing can stop you except your own disbelief.

Any fear, doubt or uncertainty about losing that weight or recovering from any other eating disorder are your own mental concoctions and have no basis in objective reality. All such negative thoughts are self-created concepts based mostly on perceived failures and baggage from the past. If you come from past mistakes or so-called failures, you are bound to repeat them. In reality, nothing more can be expected. If you come from the clear, unencumbered, open-minded present, your future mind/body is yours for the defining and asking.

Key Points and Principles:

1. That, overeating is a *subconscious habit* where the body controls the mind instead of the mind controlling the body (mind over matter).

2. That mind-body change is predicated on *self-image*, not logic or intellect.

3. That you change your self-image by *convincing* the subconscious mind, via affirmation and repetition, that you've *already* reached your goal weight.

4. That you have to be happy and content *before* you can achieve your goal.

5. That to prevent the goal-blocking stress of emotional

desire, you proceed toward your goal with the firm conviction that you've *already* achieved it.

6. That your primary motivation for achieving your goal must be *freedom and self-control* – power over your own life.

7. That you proceed toward your goal with *patient and confident perseverance* instead of mental willpower.

8. That the law of your subconscious mind *must* give you what you want; so believe without a shadow of doubt, fear, impatience or uncertainty that your goal is achieved.

9. That thinking and feeling anything negative about yourself whatsoever is absolutely false and self-created.

10. That all doubt, fear, impatience and uncertainty can be neutralized or removed from your psyche by simply keeping a conscious *distance* from them.

CHAPTER 4
VISUALIZING YOUR FUTURE

"Believing is seeing!"

Visualizing Results Is Key To Realizing Results

Visualizing is the secret to weight loss success because of three facts: one, your subconscious mind "thinks" in pictures not words; two, the subconscious is the part of your mind that drives your behavior – including your eating behavior; and three, the subconscious doesn't know the difference between something real and something vividly imagined. Whatever goal picture you consistently think about will drive your actions to exactly duplicate that picture.

Losing weight naturally and effectively is a creative process in that it uses the *imagination*. Nothing in the world is created without first being imagined. The visualization process is essential because mind-body change is predicated upon *self-image*. Determined by it.

Whether you want to write a book, start a business, invent a new product or lose weight, you have to visualize the end result first. The clearer the image the more likely you'll succeed. Clarity, like perception, is *everything*.

As your mind is a desiring machine, it's also a creating machine. You couldn't have that desire to lose weight within you unless you also had the means of fulfillment within you as well. They are two sides of the same reciprocal mind. In order for your subconscious to fulfill your desire, it needs a clear *picture* of the finished product. It has to see with complete clarity and certitude exactly what it's supposed to create.

You Have To See It Before You Can Create It

In other words, you'll need a model or archetype to emulate and replicate. For the subconscious mind, seeing is believing and accepting. If you can picture it, you virtually have it. The rest is just process, just follow-up. Before you can *physically* produce that better mouse trap you have in mind, you have to put on paper a minutely-detailed diagram of it – just as you would if presenting a new invention to the patent office for approval. – Except in this case, you're presenting it to your subconscious for approval, acceptance and fulfillment.

You want to draw a vivid mental picture of yourself at your proposed weight and keep it in the forefront of your mind. Memorialize it. You want to stamp this image onto your subconscious memory bank – superimpose it over the current image of yourself. Incorporate it – as I mentioned earlier.

This is how a "method" actor gets into her role. She

becomes her role by convincing herself, through her imagination, that she "really" is the character she's going to play. Then, when the director says "Action!" the actor plays the character perfectly because she programmed her subconscious mind that way.

Consciously or unconsciously, all the great athletes do the same. They first visualize making the perfect movement, shot or swing, then perform exactly how they pre-imagined it. The great golfer's ball doesn't land in bunkers or traps because in the visualization of the swing, they don't exist.

In the same way, you want the subconscious to *believe* that you already have the body you want. You have to *convince* it! It will then proceed to affect all systems to coincide with that vision. It will affect the serotonin, endorphin, cortisol, metabolic and hormonal levels and speeds, etc. to facilitate the creation of that body.

Along with the appropriate physiological changes, it will also inform your conscious mind when you've eaten the correct amount of food – bringing about satiety on amazingly smaller amounts of food than usual. It will make you more discriminating as to the quality, freshness and naturalness of food. It will make junk food and "comfort" food unappealing. It will diminish or end between-meal craving. It will facilitate digestion, etc. The output of the subconscious mind will perfectly reproduce the input to the degree the input is specific and the image is vivid. Just as overeating began in the mind and spread to the body, so the correction begins in the mind and spreads to the body.

The "Self-Esteem-First" Principle

Reality is whatever you think or imagine it is, so think of

this new body as the real you – as real and present as the air you breathe; while your past body is not real in the sense that it doesn't express or fulfill the real you. Just because that old body is not really *you* doesn't mean you should dislike it. If you dislike your body or hold yourself in low esteem because of it, you'll *never* control your appetite and lose that weight – because you're living under a false premise. Your old mind-body is not at fault. It's the *effect* of something, not the cause of something. Your old mind-body is totally innocent.

This is why unconditional love and acceptance of your current self and body is prerequisite to achieving your goal just as happiness-first is prerequisite. Acceptance allows and empowers change while fat-like rejection sticks to you like a magnet. Accepting your body and yourself just as they are is the first element on the ladder of change. This is called "living life on life's terms." It's living in reality. You can't change the world but you can change your attitude and response to it. "You can't control the wind, but you can adjust the sails."

Love and accept yourself with all your heart, soul, mind and strength, and never doubt yourself for an instant. Again, doubt all your doubts. There are no accidents in the universe. You had to go through all you went through in order to come to this final stage of freedom and recovery.

The Buddha said, "You can search throughout the entire universe for someone who is more deserving of your love and affection than you are yourself, and that person is not to be found anywhere. You yourself, as much as anybody in the entire universe deserve your love and affection."

Mirror, Mirror, On the Wall

Many times daily, practice picturing yourself at your goal weight and mood. If this is difficult for you, then use a photograph of you when you were the size you want to return to. Or use a photo of a celebrity whose body you can use as a guideline. If you have photo-editing software on your computer, place your head on that body. If not, just cut and paste your head onto the body. Put copies on your refrigerator, closet and all your mirrors.

You're changing your mind and that new mind is now changing your body, and you fully allow and accept this change. You accept this new self-image as the true you. Accept that you've moved onto a higher and leaner plane of existence and consciousness. You're no longer stuck in that emotion-driven body or that false idea of yourself.

You now see yourself as a thinner person sees herself. You conduct yourself as a thinner person conducts herself. You live as a thinner person lives. You think and feel as a thinner person thinks and feels. You act and speak as a thinner person acts and speaks. You eat as a thinner person eats. You face life as a thinner person faces life.

Making Your Goal-Weight Decision

The creative process begins with a goal. In this case, your *goal weight*. Lily Tomlin said, "I always wanted to be somebody, but I should've been more specific." That's a humorous observation – and true because the subconscious mind requires that your goal be *specific*. Only when the goal is clearly defined, can the subconscious begin to process your order. Specificity is a necessary factor in *convincing* your subconscious that you've *already* arrived, that that's who you "really" are right here and now. Just as you can't feed approximate numbers into your home computer, so you can't to your subconscious computer.

What's the correct or ideal weight for you based on your personal experience and research. It must be an exact, whole number like 135 pounds. It can't be *about* 135. "About" doesn't compute for the subconscious. And it can't be a weight *range* such as "between 155 and 165 pounds." That won't compute either.

The number must be realistic and based on your age, health, physical conditioning, Body Mass Index (BMI), how long overweight, advice from a health care professional, etc.

Doing The Math

Let's say you determine your correct or ideal weight to be 135 pounds, and your present weight is 178 pounds. That means you want to lose exactly 43 pounds. The next step is to determine exactly how many pounds per week you want to lose, and that'll give your *Goal Date*.

Again, all numbers should to be wise and feasible. They have to be "okay" with your conscious mind or your subconscious may "balk" at it. If you're at all uncomfortable about a particular number, change it to one that you are comfortable with.

Let's say that, based on past experience, three pounds per week is doable. Dividing 43 by 3, you get a target date of 14 1/3 weeks – which you can round off to *15 weeks*. Note that date on your calendar and journal, and as you enter your daily weight, you'll have a clear picture of your progress.

Keeping It To Yourself

A very important part of the creative process is to not tell anyone about this project. The only exceptions would be your coach, doctor or an exercise or weight-loss buddy. Blabbing to everyone in the office about your weight-loss ambition and the method you're using will dilute, scatter and drain creative energy. Keeping it to yourself keeps it focused, concentrated and sacred.

What has this to do with detachment? By virtue of following an exact plan, with exact numbers you, in effect, *remove* your old mind, self-image and false beliefs – with all its doubts and fears, from the decision-making process. And to remove yourself is to detach yourself.

What you're doing is putting yourself on automatic pilot – which is how you've operated in the past; the difference now is that you're *not* on overeating-autopilot, you're on losing-weight-autopilot. You're eating now from empowered free-will instead of unconscious compulsion. See the difference?

Internalizing Your Goal

Remember that the whole purpose and idea of any affirmation, mantra or decree is to *convince* the subconscious that something is true for you right now (even if it really isn't). In this case, it's to convince it that your goal weight is your *current* weight. We use the word *"goal"* when communicating with each other, but when communicating with your subconscious, you don't call it *goal* weight; you call it, think it, feel it, believe it – your *present moment* weight.

Your goal has to as if percolate through the hindering, "logical," insecure, part of your mind, the part that fears change, fears leaving its comfort zone. Think of the logical mind as a security guard on constant alert. It wants to "protect" you from entering the door to the frightening, subconscious unknown. But its error is that that's exactly the door to your appetite-controlling, body-changing power.

Here's a simple visualization exercise you can use to great effect: First you need to relax your body and quiet your mind.

Relaxing The Body

Gently close your eyes and take three, long deep breaths. Relax you body by simply telling each muscle group in turn to feel heavy and relaxed, and they will do so. Focus on the back of your eyelids and tell all the tiny little nerves and muscles around the eyes to relax. Now focus on the face muscles, telling them to relax and smooth out. Then tell the jaw muscles to go loose and limp. Tell the neck and shoulder muscles to be heavy and relaxed. Then arms, hands and fingers – all the way to the fingertips. Then tell the abdomen to be heavy and relaxed, then the thighs and calves, then the ankles, feet and toes.

Quieting The Mind

Detachedly focus on your breathing in and breathing out. Notice the transition points between the in and out breaths and the out and in breaths. Your breathing is becoming smooth and regular. Now begin counting each in-breath and each out-breath from one to ten over and over again until your mind has become silent and still. In a few minutes, you'll find yourself in a drowsy state similar to when just waking in the morning or when just on the verge of falling asleep. That's when your robotic security guard is most down and your mind is open and receptive to change.

Now imagine yourself sitting comfortably alone in a theater, or perhaps it's your private home theater. And in front of you is a huge movie screen. The screen lights up and you see and hear yourself, after a shower, standing on a white digital scale. The scale reads that your current and target weight is _____ pounds! You want to double check the reading, so you step off the scale for a moment then step back on to get a second reading. Yes, it's true. You now weigh _____pounds! See this clearly, for this is the weight you are and the weight you'll easily remain for the rest of your healthy, happy life.

You watch and hear yourself repeating over and over again, both softly aloud and silently to yourself, "I now weigh _____ pounds!" You're repeating it again and again. You're repeating it *believing it's true* for you right now! You keep repeating it as you dry and comb your hair. You see yourself repeating it as you get dressed for work. Repeating it during breakfast. Repeating it many times driving to work, many times at work. You see yourself repeating it until a point comes when you virtually believe it. A point when you sense that you have it. You subconscious has it!

You now see and hear yourself in a collage of scenes and situations throughout the day – looking the way you'd like to look – with the weight off those parts you'd like the weight off. See yourself at the clothing *size* you desire. This is the new and improved you. The *real* you. Someone who is slimmer, toned and fit. Just the way you want to be.

You watch yourself in that black suit you haven't been able to get into in many, many years. The one you've been saving for this moment. You feel the smooth, soft material against your skin. The smell of that fine silk is delightful.

The scenes change rapidly now and you watch your new self out shopping at the mall and notice heads turning to have a second look at you. See your confident and serene self at work – clothes hanging loose and comfortable. Co-workers looking at you a little differently. They don't quite know what you have, but they like it and want it for themselves. See yourself exercising at the gym or jogging in the park – and loving it. See yourself at a social event, vibrant and alive, laughing with friends, etc. This slimmer you is the real you. There's no longer an elephant in the room or in the mind.

Feeling Now The Way You'll Feel Then

What is that feeling that you're now experiencing and exuding? It's pure joy, isn't it? Pure pleasure! Total contentment, confidence, satisfaction and fulfillment!

To further help conjure up that feeling of pleasure and contentment, use another technique of the "method" actor. Look back over your life to a time or situation when you remember feeling immense happiness. Perhaps, for example, when you rode your first bicycle, or when you graduated high school or college, or fell in love, or got married, had your first child, got a promotion, or hit the lottery, etc. Then every time you envision your goal body, affix to it that joyful memory. Emotionalize that image. Replay this happy picture frequently – especially at meal times. Practice being happy all the time no matter what, because that's your true nature. Practice will bring you to realize it.

This "feeling-now-the-way-you'll-feel-then" is part of the "Self-Esteem-First" and the "Happiness-First" principles I mentioned earlier. You want to fill that picture with light, love and gratitude. You feel good about your life now. You feel finally free and in control of it now. And this makes you happier than you've known yourself to be in a long, long time. And holding that super-clear, slimmer, joyful image as a creative foundation, you can now begin transforming it into physical reality.

Do remember how the subconscious mind works: if you "think" all this will be difficult, it *will* be difficult. So don't indulge the idea it'll be difficult. Virtual effortlessness is an integral part of how this law works. Stress, strain and anxiety contradicts the law. This is a perfectly normal and routine procedure. The immense inner power that you possess is perfectly "normal." And any sincere person can do it.

Key Points and Principles:

1. That losing weight is a creative process in which your goal body must be visualized in vivid, minutest detail.

2. That you must feel *now* the way you'll feel when you've reached your goal.

3. That your goal must be *internalized* to be effective.

4. That you can internalize goals, subgoals and affirmations by constant repetition while the body is relaxed and the mind is still.

5. That you must love and respect yourself and your body as they are *now*, before you can achieve your goal.

6. That the key to actualizing your goal is to *convince* yourself (your subconscious self) that your future body is your present body.

7. Be realistic, conservative and exact in setting your goal weight and the number of pounds per week you plan to lose.

8. Don't tell anyone about your plan except those closest to you.

CHAPTER 5
MOVING YOUR BODY

"Fifteen-minutes a day! Give me just this and I'll prove I can make you a new man." – Charles Atlas

Let's Get Physical

So far, you've learned the specific Method or technique for overcoming the overeating habit. Then you've learned how to plan your meals and eat accordingly, then how to change your self-image, and how to picture your future body. Now we'll add *physical exercise* to your comprehensive, mind-body-spirit, new lifestyle package.

I'll come right to the point: if you don't do any physical exercise, your chances of getting slimmer are going to be very slim. Remember that this is not a pill, a stomach-stapling, or any quick fix fantasy; it's a reality-based plan of disciplined *action* – which is the only thing that works long term. All you have to do is make it a habit. Remember that good habits are just as addictive as bad habits.

The "One Day At A Time" Principle

The idea of doing something "for life" may sound a little

daunting – especially if you haven't yet habituated yourself to exercise and experienced the joy and power of it. To this end, it'll be helpful to not think in terms of a lifetime commitment, but to a *daily* commitment; a "one day at a time" approach mentioned earlier. You can practice all the steps in this Method just one day at a time. You can do anything for just one day. You can stand on your head for just one day. So, again, build an imaginary brick wall around your day and live your whole healthier, happier, thinner life within it.

Commitment to regular physical activity is more important than the intensity of the workouts. Choose exercises you're likely to enjoy – ideally ones that are part of a sport or hobby like Tennis, Golf, Ballroom dance, etc. Progress slowly. Remember, it's not necessary to be exhausted to lose weight, and it's never too late to start exercising.

Making A Commitment

Making the decision to lose weight and become healthier is a big step to take. It's helpful to put your commitment in writing – in the form of a contract with yourself. You've already "contracted" to lose a specific amount of weight by a specific date, in a specific way. Now you want to commit to a specific, well-thought-out exercise routine that works for you. It can be as simple or comprehensive as you'd like.

As the nature of the mind is to be still, the nature of the body is to move. The less the body moves the more muscles atrophy, lose tone and flexibility. Unexercised muscle groups attract fat like a magnet as metabolic rate slows and prevents the burning of that fat. Energy and vitality levels lower, causing feelings of lethargy, lack of enthusiasm, apathy, mental and physical sluggishness, etc. One part of you drags down another part of you.

Physical activity works just the opposite – it improves the quality and character of every area of life. You think better, feel better, function better and look better. Scientifically established benefits include the following: Your heart, lungs and circulatory system become stronger. Blood pressure drops. Pulse rate slows down. Red blood cells increase. Energy increases. Digestion improves. Bowels function better. Appetite is brought into line with your body's needs. Weight loss is accelerated. Libido increases. Stress is reduced. Depression reverses. The level of high-density lipoproteins (HDL) increases – which help to keep fat from building up in the arteries.

*The Physical-Activity Lifestyle

Now that you understand how important physical activity is to your health in general and weight loss in particular, the next step is incorporating it into your life. Do not feel overwhelmed by all this. It will be easier than you might think. In fact, you probably already are physically active and don't even know it. If you don't like to exercise right now, don't worry. Exercise is just one aspect of physical activity.

See if a friend would like to join you in your quest to lose weight and become more active. Things are a lot easier and more fun when a friend is involved too. Call your local Parks and Recreation Department, YMCA, or community organization to find out if they offer any programs or classes that may interest you. Many community centers and local colleges offer a variety of dance classes, exercise classes, yoga, aerobics, Tai Chi, cycling clubs, tennis lessons, swimming lessons, etc. Locate parks, and walking trails in your area. Local malls sometimes have walking clubs as well. It's a good place to go when the weather is bad.

Plan for the Week

Keep an activity journal. The journal can be separate from your eating journal or they can be combined. List all of the activities you have done or plan to do each day. A journal will help you track your progress and set goals. What has an exercise plan to do with detachment? Again, a plan removes personal discretion from the decision-making process. Track your exercise time and progress just as you record your meals. It helps you set your activity goals and stay on course. Before you know it, you'll be able to do at least 3 hours of moderate-level activities each week.

Be consistent in your program. Do it regularly every chosen day at the same time. This way you'll become psychologically and physiologically accustomed to the routine. Eventually your workout will become as habitual as showering. Don't skip more than one day. It's much too easy, particularly in the beginning, to go back to your old ways of sedentary, fat-storing, non-activity. Learn to love it and look forward to it every day with joyful anticipation. Hold the attitude that a day without exercise is like a day without sunshine.

Setting Realistic Goals

Set some short-term exercise goals and reward your efforts along the way. Focus on two or three goals at a time. Effective goals are specific, realistic, and forgiving. For example, "Exercise More" is not a specific goal. But if you say, "I will walk 30 minutes, Monday, Wednesday and

Friday for the first week," you are setting a specific and realistic goal for the first week.

Small changes every day can lead to big results. Look for progress not perfection. Also remember that realistic goals are *achievable* goals. By achieving your short-term goals one day at a time, you'll feel good about your progress and be motivated to continue. Setting unrealistic goals will only leave you feeling defeated and frustrated.

Being realistic also means expecting occasional setbacks. Setbacks happen when you get away from your plan for whatever reason – maybe the holidays, longer work hours, or another life change. When setbacks happen, get back on track as quickly as possible. Also take some time to think about what you would do differently if a similar situation happens, to prevent setbacks. When you feel like giving up, remember why you held out so long in the first place.

Everyone is different – what works for someone else might not be right for you. Just because your neighbor lost weight by taking up running, doesn't mean running is the best option for you. Try a variety of activities – walking, swimming, tennis, or group exercise classes to see what you enjoy most and can fit into your life. These activities will be easier to stick with over the long term.

The Basic Physical Exercise Program

A well-rounded program of physical activity for weight loss will include *aerobic exercise, strength training exercise, and flexibility training*. These three types of exercise need not be done in the same session. Create a pattern or routine that you're comfortable with, that you'll stick to, and that fits into your schedule.

Aerobic Activity

Aerobic activity is anything that increases your breathing and heart rate. It involves continuous, rhythmic movement of large groups of muscles to strengthen your heart and lungs. In general, you should aim to do moderate-intensity activity for a minimum of 30 minutes, five days a week, or vigorous-intensity activity for 20 minutes, three days a week. You don't have to do the entire 20 or 30 minutes in one session to enjoy the benefits. For example, you can add up your activity by doing three sessions of 10 minutes or more.

It's better to exercise for a shorter period of time than not at all. Typical aerobic exercises include *walking* – which you can do at your own pace then increase to a more brisk, deliberate speed. *Stair climbing:* Climb stairwells or use a stair-climbing machine. *Bicycling:* On the road or in the home or gym. *Jogging* burns a lot calories in a short amount of time. Start out slow and build up. Start by alternating walking with jogging. Don't increase mileage too quickly. *Swimming* puts less stress on joints and bones, and combines strength training, flexibility, and aerobic activity. *Dancing* is a great moderate-intensity activity and is lots of fun. Wear appropriate shoes and clothing. If you throw on a ragged T-shirt or sweats, it's not very inspiring for your workout. Start slowly. If you're sore or tired, give yourself extra recovery days. Remember that exercise, like happiness, is a journey, not a destination.

Strength Training

Strength-building exercises not only burn calories, they increase muscle mass. They also increase your calorie-burning metabolism – which can stay elevated for up to 48 hours after you've finished your exercise session. Strength training includes working with weights, doing calisthenics (sit-ups, push-ups, crunches, etc.), or any other resistance exercise. It targets specific body parts, making your muscles work against extra weight. Over time, the muscles become bigger to meet this demand. It can mean stronger bones, tendons, and ligaments; firmer, toned muscles; and a better sense of your body.

Eventually you can build up to 8 to 10 exercises per session that involve the major muscle groups. Do 8-12 repetitions of each exercise at least twice a week, with at least 1 day between activity sessions to allow muscles to recover. You can start with simple equipment such as 2- to 15-pound hand weights. Or use resistance bands made of strong, flexible elastic – available at sporting-goods stores. These bands can help strengthen arm and leg muscles.

Flexibility Training

Flexibility is stretching. It's the nudging of your physical boundaries. Building flexibility keeps you limber by lengthening your muscles, tendons, and ligaments. It may also decrease your risk of injury, and help you recover faster from injuries. It can help with improved freedom of movement, better posture, and increased physical and mental relaxation. After your warmup and after you finish your activity, stretch to help your muscles recover from what you've just done. Start slowly with each stretch and take deep breaths. Try to hold the stretch for 10 to 30 seconds. Don't bounce. If you feel any pain, it may be a sign you're doing too much. A few stretches after you've been sitting or standing for a while also can help you feel more energized. Some quick stretches you can try include: hamstring stretch, groin stretch, triceps stretch, hip stretch, thigh stretch, and upper arm and chest stretch. Check the Internet for free and low-cost videos of these stretches.

Yoga practice is the ultimate in flexibility training. Yoga is a combination of a set of physical and breathing exercises coupled with meditation. You can take a Tai Chi or Yoga class or buy or rent training videos. Yoga is a system of exercises to promote mind and body control. For centuries, yoga has been prescribed as moving medicine for the immune system.

Yoga has been reported to lower stress hormones that compromise immunity, while stimulating the lymphatic system to purge toxins and bring fresh, nutrient-oxygenated blood to each organ to help ensure optimum functioning. It is universally accepted for six thousand years that Yoga is highly beneficial in controlling the appetite and between-meal cravings, increasing metabolic rate, relieving stress and can help you get rid of excessive fat.

Recreational and Physical Activity

Along with Aerobics, Strength, and Flexibility exercises, you'll also want to be involved in some kind of both recreational activity – 2-3 days per week, and general physical activity – almost daily.

There are numerous activities that can be worked into your day that do not involve going to the gym, or an aerobics class. For example, walking is a very beneficial exercise most anyone can do. Do it with a friend, find a local trail. Park as far away from your destination as possible and walk. If you live in town, walk to do your errands. Take a walk during your lunch break. Walk your dog, walk the beach, walk the mall, walk to errands. Take the stairs whenever you can. Avoid elevators and escalators. If you work on the 20th floor, take the elevator to the 15th floor and walk the last five flights.

Take up a sport. Call your local parks and recreation department and find out about local softball, basketball, racket sports, soccer, etc. Jump Rope. Play Games. In-line skate, swim, bicycle, tap dance, belly dance, jazz, social and Ballroom dance. Take advantage of classes being offered in your community and have a great time while you're at it.

Try some of these outdoor activities: Gardening is strenuous work. Get outside and play in the dirt. Use a hand mower on the lawn instead of a riding mower. Go hiking, canoeing, sailing, surfing. Wash and wax your car. Clean your house. Vacuuming, mopping and dusting can be a good workout. Do simple stretching and calisthenics exercises at your desk. Do anything that gets you up and moving, and most important, have fun. Think of it this way: You get leaner and leaner every time you move your body.

Pick an activity that's easy to fit into your life. Do at least 20 minutes of physical activity at a time. Choose aerobic activities that work for you. These make your heart beat faster and can make your heart, lungs, and blood vessels stronger and more fit. Also, do strengthening activities which make your muscles do more work than usual.

How many times a week you should be physically active is up to you, but it is better to spread your activity throughout the week and to be active at least three days a week. Do a little more each time. Once you feel comfortable, do it more often. Then you can trade activities at a moderate level for vigorous ones that take more effort. You can do moderate and vigorous activities in the same week.

***Key Points and Principles:**

1. Commit to a physical exercise regimen you can live with for life.

2. Plan your exercise routine in advance.

3. Keep a journal of your exercise goals and achievements.

4. In general, exercise 20 to 60 minutes a day, 3 to 5 days a week.

5. Do moderate-intensity *Aerobic Exercises* at least 3 hours a week, or vigorous-intensity for 75 minutes a week.

6. Do *Strength Exercises* at least twice a week: 8-12 reps of 8-10 exercises.

7. Do *Flexibility Exercises* for 15 minutes at least 3 days a week – 3-4 repetitions of each stretch, holding each for 10-30 seconds.

8. Do *Recreational Activities* 2-3 days a week: swim, dance, bicycle, tennis.

9. Do some kind of *Physical Activity* almost daily for at least 20 minutes: walking, housecleaning, gardening, car washing.

*Though the exercise routines described in this chapter conform to those recommended by the *American College of Sports Medicine* (ACSM), they may not be suitable for everyone; therefore, it's important to consult with a physician or health care professional before starting any new exercise program – especially if you've been sedentary for a long time.

CHAPTER 6
CONTROLLING YOUR EMOTIONS

*"Control your emotions or they will
control you and your body!"* – WFM

Emotional self-control is about keeping a respectable distance from all that you see, hear, think, feel and do. It's the enlightened attitude of seeing all things as equal – not being affected by one thing more than another. This is the attitude of mind that gives you the unprecedented clarity and power necessary to almost effortlessly achieve your weight loss and maintenance goals for life.

How clearly you see a thing depends on how poised and relaxed (centered) you are. When relaxed, you know what you're doing, and only do what you know. Things then fall into place for you without stress or strain, and your weight-loss is achieved as a matter of course. But when you're disturbed or excited about something painful *or* pleasurable, the opposite happens. You lose your objectivity and *think* you know what you're doing rather than *know* you know. Self-control then becomes an effort and a struggle. Things don't go as planned and you experience frustration and disappointment as a result.

The Vicious Circle

Let's look at, not only how emotional stress affects your ability to see clearly, but also how it sets off a chain reaction process by which the problem is perpetuated indefinitely, and without your even being aware of it. Have you ever been so sure of something only to find you were totally wrong about it? Wasn't it bewildering? Maybe it was a personal or business decision or idea, or the choosing of a financial investment or marriage partner or weight loss program; you had considered everything so carefully. You had no doubt it was right, that it would work – then it crashed and you wondered what went wrong.

This is what happened: Instead of basing your decision on matters relating to the issue in and of itself, you became excitedly or tensely involved in it. Such involvement affected your ability to remain impartial or centered. Instead of seeing all sides of the situation dispassionately in order to make a fair and wise judgment – you influenced it. You took it *personally* instead of neutrally. Your "personal" involvement contaminated the decision-making process.

Your decision wasn't based on fact, but on the influential sway of your own personality. You colored the decision. Interfered with it. You unconsciously manipulated it to coincide with how you perhaps would've *liked* it to be, or how you believed it should, would or could be.

In other words, the decision was *personally biased*, causing the outcome to be inevitably different than the way you envisioned it – different meaning negative, and negative meaning stress. The problem is perpetuated when we carry residual tension from past situations to the present, insuring it too will result negatively.

On a short-term basis, it's like a cartoon character upset over a flat tire and reacting by kicking it and stubbing his toe. In angry reaction he punches the fender and fractures his hand, then begins to scream obscenities, is arrested for disorderly conduct and put in a straightjacket. Or more commonly, it's like resentment over a bad golf stroke, and carrying that resentment over to negatively affect the next play, and the next, until your whole game is off, which would throw your whole day off. And if we extrapolate this cause and effect cycle, your whole week, month, and life would be off.

Other examples would be fear of dogs because of being bitten as a child; fear of starting a new business venture because of a past failure; fear of closeness or openness in a relationship because of a past hurt; fear of committing to a new weight -management program because of past disappointments, and so on. Thus are we involved in a three-way, chain reaction process where one, being stressed causes us to not see clearly what we're doing; two, not seeing clearly brings about a negative or undesired outcome; and three, the undesired outcome produces stress, which makes us not see clearly what we're doing all over again.

In a circle or cycle there's no difference between the beginning and the end; they are the same point. The way it works physically is the way it works mentally and emotionally. Whenever you enter the moment tensely, you set events into motion which will bring about tension in the end. If you're in error going in, you'll be frustrated coming out; if correct going in, you'll be satisfied coming out. What goes, comes; what gives, gets. The end is always a mirror reflection of the beginning. The very state of mind or body you're in right now is the one you'll return to when all is said and done. Your future body and eating behavior is nothing more than a projection of your present state of mind.

This is the basic principle, by the way, of how some fortune-tellers "read" whether upcoming circumstances will be favorable for you. To the degree you appear calm and composed, you could expect a positive outcome, but to the degree you appear conflicted or nervous, the opposite is indicated. – Things will probably not go well, so you'd be advised to not make any important personal or business decisions at that time.

Changing The Beginning

The remedy becomes this: Change the beginning. Change the present. Willingness to change is the first step on the road to relaxation and appetite-control. "If nothing changes, nothing changes." And the thing to change is this: Enter each moment the way you want to come out of each moment – happy, content and free, regardless of what happened a second ago or twenty-years ago. This is the essence of the law of detachment.

Think of life as constantly cyclical, or as an infinite series of circles. Each circle is a new present-moment of unlimited possibilities; one you've never experienced before nor ever will again. You begin each present-moment cycle *knowing* and *expecting* that it will return full circle with the exact fruit with which it was germinated. Negative returns negative, positive returns positive.

Changing Your Attitude

Overcoming overeating is a process of changing your perspective from the self-centered way you habitually ate and lived to a more neutral way. Life is not all about you, personally. It never was and never will be. It's also not happening *to* you; it's just happening. Period. That rude clerk wasn't insensitive to you, *personally*; he just happened to be in that state of mind, and you just happened to be handy. And that half-glass of water isn't about optimism or pessimism; it's just a half glass of water. The personal view is an unreal, powerless *opinion or concept;* while the neutral, detached, universal view is a *fact*. Intelligence is not what you "think," it's the relaxed, impersonal, objective, matter-of-fact way you look at things – especially food-related things. It's this matter-of-fact viewpoint that allows you to see your overeating with such extraordinary clarity that fear, doubt and uncertainty are naturally eliminated, and all of your actions and responses become perfectly appropriate, effortless and effective.

Being detachedly centered, is nothing more than common sense, and although not so common, it's your natural and original state of being. It's who and what you really are. It's the way you were before you allowed the pressures and influences of the world excite you off balance and out of control. Becoming centered is to regain that lost balance, and along with it, your lost beauty, dignity, joy, power and freedom.

Regaining Control

Let's look at how taking life personally distorts your perception of reality, and in the process causes you to lose control of yourself; that is to say, causes your reactions to be controlled by people, places and things outside of you. Self-centeredness is a form of paranoia in the sense, for example, that those who disagree with us, we tend to feel disagree with us *personally,* so we become upset or resentful. Conversely, we're inclined to feel that those who agree with us, agree with us *personally* – so we get a swelled head instead. Disagreement frazzles us; affirmation flatters us. One drags us down, the other lifts us up.

Self-centeredness causes music to affect us similarly. We tend to take it personally or identify with it so that depending on the arrangement and tempo, it can sentimentally sink us into melancholy or stir us to cheeriness and optimism. It's due to this emotional swaying power of music that most commercial media are produced in the form of musical jingles. The "catchy" tunes influence our feelings and effectively hypnotize us into accepting or sympathizing with whatever product, person or idea is being sold. We act primarily according to how we *feel.* If our feelings can be externally controlled, then our actions and what we buy or believe can be externally controlled – and then we fully believe that it was our own decision.

The Power of Suggestion

Hypnosis is a simple two-step procedure of first getting the subject's total attention, then planting a suggestion – which is then likely to be accepted. For example, if you were asked to concentrate on *not* thinking of an elephant, you'd *have* to think of an elephant in order to process that request. So, in effect, your thinking was "controlled" by that person. Another example of hypnosis would be that of a tourist in Manhattan staring up at the top of a skyscraper, and passers by seeing him look up, stop to look up too. Soon there's a crowd looking up. It's almost irresistible to *not* look up. That's the power of suggestion.

Through the medium of television, our attention is gained through the excitement or stimulation of the senses (sensationalism). Through the sense of sight, our attention is captured by rapid-fire scenes of beautiful young people frolicking on the beach. And through the sense of hearing our attention is held by the musical jingles and loud, fast-talking salespeople or cartoon characters. Without such sophisticated entrancement techniques we'd be more likely to see the product as it *really* is, rather than as we are being led to *imagine* or *believe* it is. We would see that the product's "image" and the actual product have little in common – that there's nothing really romantic or exciting about a soft drink, for instance, that may consist of nothing more than gas, chemicals, sugar and impure tap water.

Such is the way taking life personally, negatively effects your life – by altering your perception of reality, and by controlling your reactions so that you're not really your own person, but a semi-conscious, easily suggestible victim of circumstances. It's no wonder you think there's something wrong with you or your body. The only thing wrong with you is your wrong response to the world. You need to trust yourself more, and the world less. The world is just doing its own thing and so must you. Remember the perception-is-everything principle. Don't let appearances decieve you. Just be a little more detached and discriminating so you're able to see through material life. Get a life of your own. Be independent of the world as well as a part of it. Be a leader of your own life; not a follower of others'. Stop thinking you need to overeat. You don't need to and it's okay not to.

Getting Indifferent

Taking life personally is seeing things one-sidedly and distortedly. You're stressed because you don't see the whole picture, and you don't because you're personally biased. The relaxed, centered point of view, on the other hand, works in the opposite. It relates to clarity of perception and tranquillity of mind. Being centered is seeing both sides of a situation with equal passion – like the pros and cons of a debate, for instance. Clarity is seeing a thing in its wholeness and completeness. Tranquillity means not being disturbed or excited by one side any more than the other. You're composed because you see the *whole* situation, and you see the whole situation because, as far as your higher consciousness is concerned, they're the same.

Being Impartial

Being centered is mentally balancing yourself between the two sides of any issue. It's being established in a position or attitude of neutrality with respect to all that you see, hear, think, feel and do, whether it's external or internal, painful or pleasurable. To be centered is like being a juror at a trial where fairness and justice depend on your ability to remain impartial. The prosecution is biased toward the state; the defense is biased toward the defendant. It's only for you, the witnessing, impartial juror, to remain detached. In order to make a right and fair judgment, you have to consider the evidence presented by both sides with complete equanimity.

Life itself is like a court trial in that getting to the truth is the whole object of it. It's to view the evidence of it, determine the facts of it, get to the heart of it. The prosecution and defense are like negative and positive thoughts and feelings. We are the impartial observers, the neutral witnesses to these thoughts and feelings. The prosecuting thought says, "You're wrong." The defending thought says, "No, you're right." One says, "Eat this," the other, "No, eat that." Which shall you believe and follow? You cannot believe either because both are biased opinions so are irrelevant, immaterial and incompetent.

Heart Versus Mind

Through maintaining a centered perspective, you rise above such internal conflict and allow the truth of a thing to become revealed and the way to go to become obvious. Whenever you have conflicted feelings about something, it's because you're looking at it one-sidely. You're somehow partial or prejudiced. If you're having mixed feelings over whether to eat that hot fudge sundae, for example, it's because your feelings want it but the mental doesn't think you should. There's a division, split or conflict, which indicates the wrong time or thing to eat at that time – not because the mind is superior in judgment to the heart, or vice versa, but because there's an imbalance operating, and whenever there's imbalance, there'll be error – and the consequent regret.

Here the heart says "Yes, a hot fudge sundae would be really good," but the mind says, "No, no. Don't do it. Think of the fat and calories. Think of how many miles you'll have to run to pay for it. Think of what a new wardrobe of large-size clothing would cost!" But deep down in the subconscious the choice has *already* been made. Sure, you'll rationalize it, intellectualize it, consider it from every possible angle, but we both know that sundae is going to prevail. It's like subjecting the sundae to a kangaroo court where it's given a "fair" trial before it's eaten.

Seeing Partially Versus Wholly

Clarity comes from seeing a situation in its *wholeness,* which comes from being centered in the middle of it. Seeing a thing wholly and completely is like the superior view the manager of a company has over his subordinates in the various departments. The manager of a hotel, for instance, is aware of *all* the various functions of a hotel's operation and how they're interrelated. The hotel is an organization with the manager centered among all functions. The front desk, housekeeping, sales, maintenance, accounting, and food and beverage departments, are all on the periphery. Each department is biased, so to speak; each seeing only its own narrow, limited *part* of the operation and virtually blind to the other parts, while the manager has a *view of the whole.*

Being centered between opposite poles is like the lifeguard who, standing still (relaxed) at the center of the beach – the point of maximum visibility, is more effective than one who moves (emotes) back and forth from one extreme end of the beach to the other. The "centered" lifeguard sees the whole beach at all times; the "biased" lifeguard sees only part of the beach at a time, while leaving the opposite part always unattended. The mind that's still sees clearly; the mind that moves sees distortedly.

The mind works like binoculars or a camera: The more still it's held, the clearer the view or sharper the image. In another sense, the mind works like a chimney and damper. When the damper (the viewpoint) is straight up and down (centered), the smoke (what you see and hear) can flow without being altered. But to the degree the damper is leaning left or right (being partial or prejudiced), it blocks the free passage of smoke. And while it's blocking it, it's also distorting it. Instead of the smoke passing directly and immediately out, it must now twist and contort itself around the damper, so the smoke now exiting the chimney is totally different (false) than the smoke that entered.

The Mind is Merely a Medium

All that you perceive must pass through the mind in order to be understood. The mind, like the chimney and damper, functions as a conduit through which information may process.

The higher subconscious mind, of itself, is not designed to *do* anything; it is only a *medium* of expression or passage. Its job is to be *the master reference point* of perception and action. It's job is to remain as centered as possible, as "straight up and down" as possible.

That's its most unobtrusive, unaffected position. It is then, in effect, not there at all, as when air currents turn a hanging mobile sideways so that it "appears" to have disappeared. As far as the smoke is then concerned, there is no damper. The smoke can now pass without interference and without its nature or character altered in the process.

You want free will. You want high-fidelity perception. You don't want what you see and hear to be affected on the way to your understanding. You want to get exactly what you see, and see exactly what you're getting. When the letter carrier delivers your mail, he doesn't open it to correct the grammar or rewrite it to make it sound better. He delivers it *as is*.

Getting Unaffected

Being centered is being relaxed, content, poised, detached, self-controlled, unaffected. To illustrate, think of yourself as a child's seesaw – just a straight board. When you're a centered seesaw, you're unaffected by the "ups" and "downs" of your life, because when a part of you goes up, the opposite part of you goes down an equal degree, so that your straightness or integrity is not violated; that is, you don't get "all bent out of shape." The weight or influence on one end cancels that on the opposite end, for a net effect on you of *zero*. And what's true physically, is true mentally and emotionally. When centered, the positive part of you cancels the negative part of you; what's pleasurable cancels what's painful, and so on with all pairs of opposites. As far as you, the unaffected seesaw are concerned, there's no good or bad, right or wrong, pain or pleasure. Such things are relative and exist only to the degree you choose to sit on that particular extreme. You're now above the relative. Now living in reality.

Being The Middleman

Being unaffected is like being in the position of a broker or middleman whose profit comes from the transaction itself, so is indifferent to the personalities of the buyers and sellers involved. It makes no difference if Mr. Pain is the buyer and Mr. Pleasure is the seller, or vice versa – Mr. Middleman still gets paid. On the other hand, if Mr. Middleman only desires Mr. Pleasure and avoids Mr. Pain, then the situation would be imbalanced. No sale could take place, and Mr. Middleman *would* be affected.

Similarly, the owner of a pari-mutual race track is

unaffected by the amounts won or lost by virtue of his middleman position. Every dollar won is balanced by a dollar lost. After deducting expenses and his profit percentage, the proceeds from the losers are equally divided among the winners. The negative effect of the winning tickets is canceled out by the positive effect of the losing tickets. The owner remains calm and content. He's indifferent to whether you win or lose; it's all the same to him. His only concern is that you play the game. For the middleman, the centered and relaxed man, there's no winning or losing; there's only the joy and profit of the transaction. Freedom from affectation then, involves cultivating an equal appreciation for *both* winning and losing, for *both* pain and pleasure.

Living Life On Life's Terms

Life is such that sometimes you win, sometimes lose. Sometimes there's pleasure, sometimes pain. Sometimes you're the buyer, sometimes the seller. They're two equal and inseparable sides of the same coin, the same mind; so being affected by one side more than the other is incompatible with reality. As life includes both, your embrace and acceptance should include both, for you *are* life. This is living on *life's* terms not on personally-biased, self-centered terms.

You, the higher you, don't even have a *preference* for winning, for pleasure, for sunshine. Emotional preferences, like emotional desire, are the very cause of the anxiety and stress that block happiness and self-control. Simply point your nose toward your weight-loss intention and assume it's already attained it. It's a done deal and virtually out of your mind. Then go about your business creatively instead of emotionally. Know your role, task or purpose at any given moment and involve yourself in it from the position of your higher, centered self. If it turns out negative, you won't be disturbed. If it turns out positive, you don't get excited – for the uncontrolled excitement of success will prevent your maintaining or repeating it.

Neutralizing Pressure

Holding a personal preference is holding a personal *pressure* – and is just as erroneous and harmful as being externally pressured. To be pressured is to be tilted off balance, which tends to bring the opposite of what you want – as in the seesaw illustration. Feeling pressure at school, for example, would disturb your concentration. Pressure from a friend or family member would estrange your relationship. Pressure at work would stifle your creativity. Pressure to produce or perform would inhibit performance. Pressure to conform would cause you to rebel. Pressure to lose weight would cause you to gain more weight. Pressure to stop a bad habit would strengthen its grip on you. Financial pressure would block your resourcefulness, and so on. The detached attitude neutralizes pressure, so you function more fully, efficiently, effectively, spontaneously, naturally and effortlessly. *You lose weight when the pressure and anxiety to lose weight are no longer there.*

Addicted To Pressure

Those who claim to operate better under pressure are really subconsciously addicted to it. The person who *needs* pressure to function is wrongly motivated. The rightly motivated person works first for the work itself, for the action itself. Success follows as a natural side effect.

But the wrongly motivated person has it backwards: He works for the side effect first – the money first, for example. He has a problem, for once he's reached his financial goal, there's no longer any "real" reason to be productive, so he must create artificial pressure through the emotional, endless pursuit of more and more expensive toys, entertainments and diversions. He spins in a circle like a mouse on a spending-to-earn, earning-to-spend treadmill. Once he arrives at each new plateau of so-called success, he crashes into the reality of the nonfulfillment and emptiness of it. He finds higher and higher mountains to climb only to end up where he began – hungry and discontent. Only if he lives long enough does he come to realize that the top is not where "it" is at; where it's at is in the journey. It's en route. It's in the infinite action – mentioned earlier. It's always in the exact spot where you happen to be standing at any given moment. The top of the self-control mountain is not a place; it's a state of mind right here and now.

Raising Your Emotional Thermostat

Being centered, along with its increased clarity, joy and power, does not necessarily come all at once, but only to the degree you can manage or control it. Obviously, if you become overly excited you're not centered any longer. That's the catch. Detachment allows awareness to increase, but as soon as it does, excitement about it immediately blocks its continuance. So you move one step forward, one step backward, either not growing at all or growing at the pace of a snail.

This up and down relaxation/excitement cycle works like a thermostat control: clarity, joy and power rise to the point of excitement – then shut off. Your task becomes raising the excitement point higher and higher so that self-control can rise correspondingly. In other words, you want to become less and less excited about more and more things. Wisdom and power, are nothing more than the ability to either enjoy or suffer without making an emotional issue of it. Feelings are just feelings, and the more relaxed and detached you are, the more above and in control of all feelings. You need less and less food to satisfy you.

Stress itself is a neutral energy but becomes negative when carried away by it, and becomes positive when kept under control, kept neutral. Being controlled is not "cold" as commonly misinterpreted. On the contrary, you not only feel the entire spectrum of human emotion, you feel it even *more* vividly, *more* passionately – but you're not excited or disturbed by it. Nothing in life should surprise you because there's simply no end to its novelty to the degree you venture from your self-imposed comfort zone.

Balance Controls And Enhances All The Personal Faculties

Balance via "keeping your distance" controls physical, mental, emotional and sensual energy so you can operate, grow and act more effectively and efficiently. Physical balance, such as pacing yourself during physical activity, controls and conserves that energy. Mental balance or stillness conserves psychic energy so you can think better. The nature of the body is to move, but the nature of the mind is to be still. If the body isn't exercised, muscles atrophy; if the mind isn't stilled, intelligence and power atrophy. Being emotionally centered is how you control painful or pleasurable feelings so you don't get carried away by either, so you don't eat over either. And being sensually centered is what allows you to be more discriminating as to the quality, quantity and character of all you see, hear, taste, touch and smell – making it virtually impossible to eat the wrong thing or at the wrong time or for the wrong reason.

Key Points and Principles:

1. That you control your emotions by feeling them from an appropriate and respectable *distance*.

2. That emotional control is experiencing good and bad feelings as just the same.

3. That emotional control is key to clarity of perception.

4. That emotional control makes you less susceptible to outside influence, suggestion and temptation.

5. That emotional control lets you see wholly instead of partially.

CHAPTER 7
KEEING YOUR DISTANCE

*"Thought, feeling and sensation are below you,
and that's where they have to be kept!"* – WFM

When centered via "keeping your distance," you're living in reality or *truth* – truth being defined here as that which exists *before* you personalize it, conceptualize it or emotionalize it. The only difference between being emotional and being relaxedly and detachedly centered is that in the one case, you're *out* of control, and in the other, *in* control.

The emotional person is scattered; the detached person is collected. The emotional person is possessed by the world; the detached is self-possessed. The emotional can be excited or depressed by anything, while the detached person isn't excited or depressed by anything. The emotional person is a slave – for whatever inflates or depresses her, owns her. The detached person is free while the emotional person is disconnected from her source and center so is easily taken over – especially by food.

The relaxed, detached person is connected to her center so is clear and confident as to when and how to eat and when and how to stop. There's no "dieting" involved. Food is no more an issue in her life than is walking and talking. She eats when hungry and stops when the hunger has passed. She's not *doing* control; she's *being* control. Being herself – her higher self. Self-controlled is who she naturally is. It's not something that has to be thought about.

The word "excite" means to *move away*. To relax means to loosen back, to be restored to a previous condition. When you're relaxing, you're "steppng back" back to your original state of effortless being – which is the state of centered relaxation. Living in non-attached freedom is living in your relaxed home, your ideal, your center of operations. Whenever you leave it, you feel discomfort; whenever you distance yourself from it, you feel at ease. Stress or excitement is what pulls you away from that center, and recovering your distance is what brings you back.

Maintaining Your Integrity

Detachment comes by degree, and to the degree you're centered via detachment, you transcend being emotionally affected or disordered by anything – including food. On a lower level, you'd be unaffected by rain or sunshine; on a higher level, you'd remain unaffected even if that rain brought you financial disaster, for example. Your essential wise and good nature wouldn't change, and you wouldn't leap from the roof of a building. Your spouse, children and dog might leave you. Your friends might be dismayed. The bank may take your home, and the Internal Revenue Service may padlock your business. You might even have to sleep in a public shelter and stand in soup lines, but none of this would uncontrollably distress you. You'd remain your calm and composed self. External conditions could not corrupt the real you, the beautiful you, the eternally poised and courageous you. – Of course, being so calm and clear you wouldn't come to such an extreme in the first place. You'd have anticipated the problem, or if not, you'd have had the creative power to make the necessary course corrections and bounce back.

The point is to become less and less affected by more and more things until you realize that nothing external can harm you; that it's only when you allow outside influences to get under your skin that you overeat; that even if you were at rock bottom you'd still be all right. You'd still survive, that you had always survived and that you always would; that there's indeed nothing to fear; that all that *appears* negative in life doesn't exist in objective reality, but is merely an illusion born of a self-centered outlook or perspective.

Living On An Even Keel

With higher degrees of unaffectedness, pain becomes less and less painful until you can't differentiate between it and pleasure. The dividing line between them diminishes until it disappears, and you're not sure whether you're supposed to laugh or cry. There are no more ups and downs. They become equal. The mountains lower and the valleys lift. Now there's only one you, not two. You've risen above all superficial distinctions of pain and pleasure, failure and success. Now there remains only joy, peace and contentment. In such a state, your mind is in order and so is your relationship with your body and your food.

Rolling With The Punches

To live in a non-personal way is to have a ball by being a

ball. A ball can't be emotionally affected because, being round, it has no sides or positions to be partial to or prejudiced against. It's equal on all sides, the same all around. It can roll with equal ease in any direction the situation happens to be slanting. A ball can't land wrong-side up or upside down because it has no such distinctions or boundaries. When you're a ball, there's only one way you can ever land – right-side up. To be centered, then, is to be a ball; to be biased, is to be a square.

Being round enables you to roll with the punches of the world. Whenever you stand flatfooted or fixed, the slightest tap will rattle your brain or tip you over. In order to be unaffected by the world, your head and the world's fist must move, not toward each other, and not away from each other either, but in the same direction at the same time – more as if you were dancing rather than fighting. Life becomes a harmonious dance, not a conflicting struggle.

Given the hardness of the world and the softness of your head, wisdom demands a response to life that's more in tune with the world. To roll with the punches is not to compete with the world, but to cooperate with it, harmonize with it. When the orchestra is playing a tango, then dance the tango, not the Watusi; when at a funeral, be somber not cheerful. When at a wedding, be cheerful not somber. You don't tell the world what to do; the world, that is, the situation, tells you what to do.

My friend Maxie lost his job as waiter-trainee as a result of not understanding this principle of rolling or floating with the situation as opposed to being self-centeredly stuck in one position: He was balancing a large tray of fruit cocktails on one hand while serving them to guests with the other, when for the third time that evening the tray and dishes tipped over and crashed to the floor. When the manager came to investigate, Maxie explained that he was holding the tray at the exact center as he was told, but that after he had served two or three, the tray just tipped over by itself.

"But didn't you keep shifting your hand to compensate for the changing distribution of weight?" asked the manager. "Didn't you keep re-centering your position?"

"No," said Maxie, "I was trained to just hold the tray at the center."

"But the point of balance isn't a *fixed* point," said the manager, "It isn't a *particular* place. If the tray were empty, yes, the point of balance *would* be the center, but the tray is not alone in the world; it lives in relationship with the dishes. So the center must be flexible to accommodate their spontaneous comings and goings. Every time a dish is removed from the tray it's a different situation, so you must move your hand to the new point of balance, the new center!"

"I didn't know you had to be an engineer to wait tables," replied Maxie.

That's when the manager politely asked Maxie to turn in his apron and leave the premises forthwith.

It's Not All About You

Self-centeredness operates under the misconception that *he* is the center of all experience, that everything revolves around *him*. In reality, the *situation* is the center, not you, personally. You're merely the actor, the player, the participant. The situation is the thing. Or in Shakespeare's words, "The play is the thing." You are nothing; the situation is everything. Again, the transaction is where the action is. Error is self-centered while detachment is situation-centered or neutrally-centered. The self-centered is full of himself, while detachment has no self. Detachment is free from his lower appetite while his ego-self is controlled by it.

Being Relaxed While Excited

You don't want to eliminate, suppress or repress emotions. That's a common misunderstanding of this principle. Emotions are integral to health, clarity and happiness. What you do want to do is *control* them. Either you control them or they control you. There are no other choices. The how is to be relaxed *while* excited – another seeming paradox. Your usual pattern is to bounce back and forth between excitement and relaxation like a ping-pong ball. Something moves you and *later* you calm down from it. Tension then calmness, then tension then calmness. Your goal is to move the excitement part of the cycle and the relaxation part closer and closer together until they overlap or occur simultaneously. You want to be composed *as* you move, like a ballet dancer who can flit freely around the stage while maintaining a graceful and dignified poise every step of the way.

Being composed and excited at the same time is a process similar to that of walking up a down escalator where excitement is at the bottom, and relaxation is at the top. In order to stay centered between them, you have to move up at the same speed as the escalator is moving down. In this way you remain still *while* moving, calm *while* excited, and is way to fully experience both the painful and the pleasurable without being negatively affected by either. When there's no discomfort, there's no reason or desire to overeat.

Getting Positive

The question becomes, what's your state of mind or feeling when you see all things with equal eyes? What's the prevailing mood when unaffected by neither pain nor pleasure? The feeling is one of *pleasure*. Why? Because whenever you're centered between opposing emotions, you automatically take on the *positive* one. When centered between doubt and confidence, you become confident; between resentment and acceptance, you become acceptant or forgiving; between guilt and innocence, you feel innocent, and likewise with all feelings. The positive always dominates with a balanced, centered attitude because it's the pole most compatible with your true nature, with reality.

Human nature is essentially positive because conscious life in and of itself is a good and positive thing. Positive in that it's whole, compete, real, perfectly ordered, perfectly controlled. So to the degree you are centered in attitude, you become whole, complete, real, perfectly ordered and controlled yourself. You become compatible with life instead of at odds with it; consequently, the positive is what you'll naturally feel and express.

This principle is like the traffic law that says that when two vehicles approach an intersection at the same time (in balance), the one on the right (the positive one) has the right of way (becomes dominant). But when your perspective is imbalanced, you block out a part of yourself like a cloud blocks the sun. So you become, in effect, un-whole, unreal, uncontrolled, disordered and stressed – and that's when you head for the refrigerator.

The sun isn't *really* gone; it's just blocked. This incompleteness or un-wholeness is felt as a negative deficiency or emptiness that you try to fill with food. Others try to fill it with sex, alcohol, gambling, shopping, etc. The thing to grasp here is that all such negativity is false. Negativity has no basis in reality. It's merely an appearance – an emotional optical illusion that's corrected when you change from a personal, self-centered angle of vision to a more neutral or universal one. Think of negativity as an empty cup that has to be filled with illicit food; when you don't have negativity, there's nothing that needs to be filled, so no need to overeat.

A Double-Barreled Centering Technique

Staying relaxed and centered is a simple procedure of knowing what your present mood is, knowing what its opposite is, then moving between them by either *rejecting both* or *accepting both*. Let's say you're feeling angry toward someone. The opposite of anger is forgiveness, tolerance or acceptance. In *rejecting* both, don't accept the perceived offense and don't resent it either. Just remain the same, calm and composed – as if nothing happened.

In *accepting* both, you resent and accept simultaneously, or as close together as possible. Here it's more obvious that nothing has changed, that you remain controlled and unaffected. So you don't have to eat over it. Or, in simpler terms, when you're angry, count to ten; when feeling depressed, start singing; when sad, start laughing; when bored, get curious; when doubtful, exude confidence, etc. Again, the subconscious mind is imaginative and creative not logical. The Method of positive living is simply to contradict out of existance anything in your mind that's not positive.

"... And The Truth Shall Make You Free."

Overlooking the offense of others is, again, based on the reality that how a person behaves is *his* problem not yours. It's not any of your "personal" (emotional) business. If a patient in an insane asylum insulted you, would you become upset? Of course not, because you'd *know* the cause of his behavior is his mental illness and not you, personally.

Knowledge of his insanity would balance out the effect of the insult so you'd remain undisturbed. Now suppose an aggressive driver dangerously cuts you off on the highway. Would you then react with anger? It would be wrong for the same reason as above – that the cause of the aggressiveness or rudeness is his problem not yours. It's a mental imbalance on his part and has nothing to do with you, personally. The appropriate responsed is to simply and safely get out his way.

The "sickness" here will of course be less obvious than in the above instance, but the difference is merely one of setting and degree – mental imbalance remains the case. You would respond appropriately but not with anger (or overeating). There's no emotional reaction to the *person,* but a composed response to the *situation.*

The difference is that in the one case, you're out of control, and in the other, in control. In one case you're self-centered, in the other, *situation-centered.* In one case you took it personally, in the other, centeredly.

It Takes Two To Tango

The rule of thumb is this: Whatever you emotionally say or do will tend to be reactive and wrong; whatever you impersonally say or do, will tend to be responsive and correct. Reacting with anger effectively makes you imbalanced too by pulling you away from your own center of poise. Through emotional reaction in general, and resentment in particular, the dis-ease of another is transferred to you. It's contagious. You complete the transaction some person, place or situation initiates. Something's being offered or suggested to you. You're being tested. Tempted. Will you accept? That's the question. It's attempting to sell you something. Will you buy?

It takes two to complete a transaction. If you react emotionally, then you become its customer, its market. You put yourself in the same league with him or it. You are playing its game, on its level, and by its rules. He or it, consciously or unconsciously, is now controlling you, hypnotizing you, exciting you, exploiting you, dominating you. You're no longer in possession of yourself; no longer your own person but have become subject to him or it. It acts and you re-act; it's the cause and you're the effected; it's the mover and you're the moved – straight to the refrigerator.

The world is like a glass windshield that has shattered into four billion interconnected people. The only difference among them is that each reflects "reality" at a slightly different angle. They're all of the same substance, but each expresses that substance according to his own unique, personal perspective. As far as higher consciousness is concerned, there are no good pieces or bad pieces, no right or wrong pieces. There are just *different* pieces. We come to realize that "reality" can't be seen with personal eyes, but only with impersonal, detached eyes.

Being Mirror-Like

The opposite of being a personality is being a medium or mirror. A mirror doesn't have any particular qualities or characteristics of its own. It simply reflects faithfully whatever is presented to it. The nature of a mirror is to be perfectly clear, for any blemish will affect the fidelity of its reflection. If it has any thoughts or beliefs of its own, then it'll no longer be an honest mirror but one that distorts everything it sees accordingly. If the mirror is to be effective, it cannot have a "self" of its own. It must be selfless; that is, it must have no opinions or concepts of its own in order to be able to see and reflect with purity and integrity.

Getting Creative

Thinking is an activity, and like desiring, it can be either emotional or creative. As a general rule of thumb, if thinking doesn't go somewhere in particular, doesn't contribute to solving a problem or achieving a conscious objective, then it's emotional. Hoping, trying, expecting, desiring, daydreaming, wishing, resenting, complaining, worrying, and the like, are emotional because they're of a negative, dead-end nature. They have no positive end. They just sit there sapping energy and giving nothing in return. Creative thought, on the other hand, leads to and coincides with productive action. It brings problems and goals to resolution. There's no waste, no fat. Each thought pulls its own weight and contributes coherently to a moment to moment or overall plan. When you control thought and feeling, they become creative, and bring goals to fruition. When thoughts and feelings control you, creativity is stifled or blocked, and you experience frustration and failure. – Relief from which is as close as your refrigerator.

The question to ask is, who's in charge here, you or your feelings? You are in control of your feelings because you can *observe* them. To be the observer is to be the controller, because the observer is *above* the things he observes; he's *superior* to them. You can objectively observe your thoughts, feelings and food issues, therefore, you can control them at will. You're not powerless over your food disorder to the degree you get above it, and you get above it by virtue of conscious detachment from all aspects of it.

The Law of Allowance

The *law of allowance* is related to the law of detachment. To allow or accept your disorder is to effectively separate yourself from it. You don't have to "do" anything in order to control your mind or your eating. No mental activity is required. All that's necessary is the indifferent observation of it. To allow your overeating *is* to control it because then you're no longer emotionally entangled in it. You're detached from it. It's under control because you've removed the *conflict* that rendered you powerless over it. Conflict itself is the impotence factor; it's the killer of personal power and self-control.

Letting Go

Letting go means dropping the idea that you can "think" yourself into control of your appetite. Descartes said, "Perhaps everything we believe is false." If we're not living in detached reality, we're living in powerless ignorance, trance or illusion. Our "thinking" gives us the false impression that we're in control. The more we "think" the more we imagine we are masters of our lives. The fact is that apart from objective, subconscious reality we are nothing; we have no *personal* control over our eating disorder whatsoever. The master of self-control said, "Of yourself (your lower, personal self) you are nothing." – You can do nothing. To the degree you're tuned with objective reality, your disorder virtually corrects itself. Your "personal" knowledge, of itself, not only has nothing to do with it, but constitutes being out of order in the first place. It's what hinders recovery.

Everything you need to know to control your appetite and unwanted habits is within you right now and always has been. You don't have to reinvent the wheel. The universe has already been thought out for you. All you have to do is tap into it, flow along with it – and detachment is the way to do it. It's the means by which to let go of your lower self – which is the controlled not the controller.

Letting go is both difficult and easy – difficult in that, without all those positions and conditions about life and food that you've wrapped yourself in, you'd feel naked and vulnerable. But nakedness and vulnerability are the whole idea; they are the very essence of freedom. To be open and exposed means you have nothing to hide, nothing to defend, and therefore, nothing to fear or be anxious about, and nothing to eat over. All fear is the fear that, of yourself, you are nothing, compounded by the fear that others will discover it. The fact is that, of your (lower) self, you really are nothing and so is everyone else.

Letting go of personal shortcomings is achieved by acknowledging them and accepting them. Then they drop by themselves. It'll be easy in the sense that you don't have to add anything to yourself, but rather, to drop things you've accumulated. We are all products of the same human condition. What you want to do now is to make the human condition a product of *you*. You do this by keeping your distance from everything that's holding you against your will, whether from the past or in the present. To hold on to something takes energy and effort, but to release a thing requires neither – you just drop it. Separate from it. Disown it. Dis-identify with it.

Imagine that you're carrying all your knowledge (fat) in a shopping bag, years and years of accumulated information and misinformation are packed into it making it a very heavy load. To hold on to this bag day in and day out takes energy and effort, but to let it go, all you have to do is relax your hand. Release your grip and the bag (the fat) falls by itself.

You Are Always Enough

If external information is so necessary to the control of your life and your appetite, then how could you ever have enough of it? Where would it end? At what point would you consider your knowledge sufficient? If there's no end to it, there can't be a beginning either; that is, if you're deficient in something right now, then you'll always be. The book that would provide the knowledge needed to cope with this moment has not yet been written. And when it is, it'll be immediately obsolete, for the situation that called for it will be gone, and the new situation will have a completely different set of variables, requiring yet another book that will also be obsolete on completion, and so on.

In other words, by depending on past knowledge to control yourself, you remain in the past yourself. You remain in a state of perpetual obsolescence. It's like being the trailer behind the car: The car is like reality, and the trailer is like the knowledge-dependent person who must always lag behind it.

The information necessary to handle this moment intelligently must come out of this moment, not out of the past – from within you, not from outside of you. Outside information is dead and gone; inside information (subconsious intuition) is alive and ever-present.

Being Empty-minded

To be prepared to move in any direction with equal ease requires a mind that's open, empty and still. A mind that contains anything at all will be restricted by those contents. Such a mind will not be able to "think on its feet" unless the questions that come up just happen to correspond with the predetermined answers it's carrying around. Which is unlikely, for reality does not conform to us; it's for us to conform to it. To have an answer without a question is just as useless as having a question without an answer.

Open-mindedness means not having any answers – or any questions either; it's being totally empty so as not to impose limits on your own intelligence or common sense. Think of that bag of positions you're carrying as full of dead information like yesterday's newspaper. Pages and pages of dead answers to questions life is never going to ask again, and each answer having the effect of limiting or diminishing you a bit. Each premeditated answer uses up some of your intelligence like a computer's random access memory (RAM) is used up, so at any given moment you're operating below speed and capacity. As you let the newspaper go when finished, so let the moment go when it's finished. Enter each new moment fresh, open, receptive. Keep your mind clear. Be ignorant like Socrates. Don't have any knowledge of your own, but be impartially interested in the knowledge of others.

Changing Your Beliefs

The law of reverse effort applies to "believing" as well as to any other activity. You tend to be the opposite of what you think or believe. If you think you know it all, you know nothing; if you think you are wise, you are a fool; if you think you are educated, you are ignorant; if you think you are great, you are common; if you believe you're the life of the party, you are a bore, and so on. "Believing," in and of itself, indicates just the opposite – that you are doubting. Belief and doubt are two sides of the same mind, so that it's impossible to have a belief about something without also having a doubt about it.

To transcend this paradox, apply the *"Double-Barreled Centering Technique."* Depending on your personality, you can either believe everything or believe nothing; doubt everything or doubt nothing. Those are the only two choices that reality offers and no split orders, substitutions or exceptions are allowed. To let go, surrender, give up, all mean the same thing: to relinquish something lower so that something higher may operate. It means dropping the narrow, limited personality so that the higher potentiality within may work in its place. The intelligent organism that you are is what you're surrendering to. When through detachment, you give *in* or give *up,* it refers to our subconscious organism. When we go to sleep, we trust it, we give up to it; so why can't we do likewise when awake as well? Why can't we not give up to it when relating to our body and our food? Stop believing that you can't.

Being a Receptacle

In order to experience the reality of recovery from overeating, you have to be receptive to it. Think of reality and yourself as two halves that join inside of you. Reality doesn't have a self or body of its own; it's "spiritual" like electricity and must live *through* you. Conversely, you don't have spirituality of your own but must live *from* it. We are merely receptacles into which this spirit may plug. Together we constitute reality; separate we exist as a powerless falsity. Just as a toaster isn't "really" a toaster until plugged into its source of power, so you aren't "really" a happy, intelligent and powerful human being unless plugged into your source of power – which is the subconscious mind.

Being Commonsensical

When you're not "thinking," you're able to make direct contact with your body. Otherwise your stomach remains at arms length like a stranger – something with which you can't be intimate or responsive to. With a receptive and detached mind, you become fused to your body. You become consciously as well as organically connected to it like the head and tail of the same animal. It's only through being so connected with your body that you can know it and respond to it intuitively and immediately. Intuition is not emotional; it is essential common sense. It's operating with a clear conscience, a conscience unclouded and undisturbed by emotionality or personality.

Common sense is the ability to notice a pattern in what's going on and to spontaneously pinpoint the significance of it without having to *think* about it. When you see a work of art, for example, you know right off whether it "works," whether you like it. It correlates with your sense of harmony or doesn't.

When listening to a piano recital and a wrong note is struck, you know it immediately, even without ever having heard the piece before or without any musical training. The same with your eating life: To the degree you're centered via detachment, you see your eating behavior with such acute clarity, that it becomes easy to stop or change it. It's only the incomplete picture of what you're doing to yourself and body that's been blocking your power to correct it.

Key Points and Principles:

1. That "keeping your distance" is the primary method of being centered, balanced and grounded.

2. That "keeping your distance" is like being the impartial juror at a trial, or the indifferent middle man in a business transaction.

3. That "keeping your distance" gives clarity and control of how you think, feel and eat.

4. That "keeping your distance" neutralizes food-related conflicts.

5. That "keeping your distance removes the emotion and conflict that renders you powerless over your appetite.

 6. That "keeping your distance" breaks the trance of unconscious overeating.

7. That "keeping your distance" is the ultimate method of self-mastery.

 8. That "keeping your distance" is the attitude that allows you to experience the ups and downs of life with equanimity.

CHAPTER 8
OVERCOMING YOUR STRESS

*"Stress is caused by taking life
personally instead of neutrally!"* – WFM

Stress is public enemy number one. It's the root cause of most every preventable disease and unwanted condition that we experience in life. It negatively affects every part of our life – our health, happiness, clarity and appetite-control power. Managing stress is prerequisite to quality of life in general and to weight management in particular, so let managing it be the number one priority in your life.

Stress-control is based on the following logic: *If feelings of discomfort trigger overeating, then stop feeling discomfort.* Here we're treating both the cause and effect of the problem – knocking the whole eating-for-comfort habit into oblivion. Negative thoughts and feelings, such as of discontent, boredom, loneliness, anger, resentment, fear, doubt, guilt, uncertainty, worry, etc., control you more than logical thinking does. If you can't control these negatives, you won't be able to control much of anything else in your life – especially your appetite.

Appetite-control *is* stress-control and vice versa. Feel your feelings fully, both the negative and the positive ones, but don't let any take you over – get under your skin. Oscar Wilde put it this way, "A man who is master of himself can end a sorrow as easily as he can invent a pleasure. I don't want to be at the mercy of my emotions. I want to use them, to enjoy them, and to dominate them."

The battle of the bulge is between impulse and restraint, desire and self-control, instant gratification and healthy delay. Resisting the impulse to eat when not hungry or to eat beyond satiety, is key to self-control. Think it through. Remember that when you choose a behavior, you choose the consequences.

Controlling Pain And Pleasure

We can greatly simplify the matter with the understanding that, in the whole world, there are only two emotions – negative ones and positive ones. For our purpose here, all other terms are academic. Names themselves don't matter; only their meaning matters. Emotion means movement; so "negative" means a backward movement – *away* from achieving your goal; "positive" means a forward movement – *toward* the achievement of your goal. But for communication purposes we'll name some of the emotions – the most important of which is *contentedness*, which I talked about in Chapter 1.

True contentedness means that if your desires are not fulfilled, it doesn't make any difference to your happiness or well-being. If it doesn't make any emotional difference whether or not you lose weight, then you've already lost that weight; if it doesn't make any emotional difference whether or not you win, you've already won. This, again, is the *law of detachment*, and is what being relaxed and centered is all about.

Contentedness means you're not deficient or lacking in anything. Nothing's missing from you. You are complete and whole. You've reached to the understanding that, as Marcus Aurelius put it, "Everything is just as it is supposed to be." You have arrived. Whether you're a dishwasher or chairman of the board, it's only your contentedness that indicates that you are free and secure; that you have overcome the world.

Contentedness is indifference to both pleasure and pain. As far as your higher self is concerned, they are the same. You, the higher you, are unchanged, unfazed by either. You remain yourself – calm, composed, indifferent. Indifference means one is no different than the other. You accept them as equals. You don't (emotionally) desire that a situation be different than it is. You are pre-established in contentment. It is one of your highest and most powerful pre-existing conditions. It's equal to bliss, deep serenity and love. *Contentedness* (acceptance) is what transcends and controls pain and pleasure of any name or nature.

Pursuing Pleasure Produces Pain

The opposite of indifference is *emotional desire*. When you desire emotional relief through food, it means you've left the state of balanced relaxation and contentment, and negative feelings will be the inevitable result.

There's nothing wrong, of course, with pleasure and gratification in and of themselves, it's the emotional *desiring* part of the equation that causes the problems. Desiring is the emotional pressure that pulls you off balance and into the negative cause and effect, vicious cycle. Craving gratification is an emotional activity, and just like physical activity it's subject to the law of reverse effort that says "All action produces an equal and opposite reaction." So that whenever you seek gratification through food, you tend to get the opposite – pain, in the form of disappointment, frustration and failure. When you emotionally seek to lose weight, you tend to gain weight.

This principle also applies if you're experiencing pleasure and try to retain or cling to it. The clinging, like desiring, causes the pleasure to change to pain. But if you are experiencing pleasure and are indifferent to it – it remains.

And the same is true of emotional discomfort. If you try to escape it, it persists, but if you experience it totally and indifferently, it changes to pleasure. Pleasure is relaxation, comfort and contentment. It indicates a state of joyous equanimity. Physical balance is the absence of physical pain, mental balance is the absence of negative thinking such as doubt or disbelief, and emotional balance is the end of stress.

When you have no cravings or desires, you are relaxed and serene. Being relaxed and pain-free is perfectly natural. The proof that it's natural lies in the fact that when you're without pain you don't notice it, but if you have a worry, a headache or a desire, you're continuously uneasy. Pleasure is the norm. Pain is the aberration. When there's no pain, you just go joyfully about your business without thinking about it. You don't notice it. Peace and joy don't need a reason, but to suffer you need guilt, doubt, fear, etc.

Enough Is Enough

Needing a reason to be happy is not natural; it indicates disease. If you need a *reason* to be happy, then you can never be happy because the illusory deficiency that seeks a reason now will always remain. As soon as you meet or are about to meet your criteria for "happiness" – immediately your seesaw of imbalance will pop up with yet another requirement, and then another. Your work is never rewarding enough. Life is never exciting enough. You never meet the "right" man or woman. You never have the money, possessions or security you think you need. You never receive enough appreciation or recognition, etc. Applied to eating, you can never get enough food to sate the discomfort or fill the void. Discontent endlessly breeds further discontent. It's like trying to stabilize a rocking canoe, as soon as you move to one side, the other side wants to tip you.

If you're looking for a *reason* to be happy, you'll always be looking. You'll remain a seeker and never a finder. Nothing will satisfy you. Everything will contain some insufficiency, some defect. Something will always be missing or falling short of the mark. If you're not content with what is at this moment, then you can't be content with what should, would, or could be either. The only choice you have, then, is to be *choiceless*. It's to live in a state of total acceptance and allowance.

Being Independently Happy

What is, is real; what should be is fantasy. Living in reality, in and of itself, is pleasing and gratifying. But living in accordance with how things should, would or could be, breeds endless frustration. If you're not happy in the rain, you can't be happy in the sun either for they are two sides of the same weather coin. In the first place, you cannot accept or reject only half a coin, and in the second place, the whole coin is irrelevant to happiness.

Happiness is not dependent on one thing or another. It's totally self-sufficient. Like life, it doesn't come *from* things but exists in and of itself. Happiness is inherent not derivative. It's free-standing. Nothing external is needed. Happiness is just the way life is whether we like it or not, and has nothing to do with rain or shine, good or bad, right or wrong, fat or lean. So we have no choice but to like it. The attitude of reality is "Love it or leave it." When you overeat or under eat, you are leaving it.

Circumstances are just the props of life; just the scenery, setting or background. The backdrop is ever changing, but the real you, the authentic, relaxed you, remain always the same. One day you wear a blue suit, the next day a gray one; one day goes well, the next doesn't. Behind the suit and aside from the fluctuations in the market, you're the same person. The real, higher you cannot change, cannot become unhappy, unrelaxed. Unhappiness is a dis-ease that doesn't occur in reality; it's something that's acquired, and we acquire it through emotionally desiring things be different from what they are right now. Life is neutral; it becomes a problem when we judge and criticize it; and it becomes joyous when lived indifferently and impersonally.

Pain Is an Imbalance Warning Signal

The purpose of physical, mental or emotional pain is to warn us that something unhealthy is going on. In health, the whole organism is working harmoniously; in disease, some imbalance or conflict is in effect, and pain is the means by which we're informed of it. If you're sitting on a hot stove, the pain would alert you to the danger. Likewise with emotional pain such as that of anxiety or resentment. It's to remind us we're desiring something inappropriate or desiring in the wrong way.

So discomfort is really a positive thing; it's a friend not an enemy. It's not the problem itself but merely the messenger. Our mistake, of course, is that we try to kill the messenger instead of the *cause* of the problem. When there's physical pain we respond quickly and decisively. As soon as we notice the stove is hot we stop touching it and are not likely to repeat the error. But emotional pain and tension are more subtle, not so compelling an emergency. So instead of seeking to understand and treat the cause, it's more expedient to just kill the messenger – which we attempt to do with various distractions, such as alcohol, drugs, sex, gambling, shopping, stock market, work, or food, etc.

Treating The Cause Not The Symptom

Treating the symptom is quick and easy, but relief, if there is any, is superficial and fleeting. We want instant gratification but the side effects are often worse than the dis-ease itself. It's like instead of getting off the hot stove, you just sat there taking aspirin and tranquilizers – or trying a different diet program. The implication of all this is that maintaining a centered perspective or attitude is not a choice but a *law*. Yes, you do have the freedom of choice – to break or obey that law. But if you choose to break it, there will be a sure penalty – like gaining weight. So, in reality, you don't have a choice. Universal law has to be obeyed. The universe is so structured that if you don't maintain an attitude of relaxed indifference to it, you'll get burned, then seek relief in food.

Success is finding your own level, your own pace. It's to not go too fast or be too ambitious, and it's to not go too slow or be stagnant. It's to remain in the middle. Centered. The world turns at a certain speed and it's for you to find that speed. It's to "go with the flow." The pain of stress will be your foolproof guide. No need to rationalize or intellectualize it. Simply notice the exact moment when the tension or craving arises, then stop being affected by the feeling or stop doing what you're doing. Change the subject.

And it's likewise while eating, notice when the hunger has abated then stop eating. When Pinocchio lied, his nose grew; when we lie or sin against our nature, our stomach grows.

Don't Desire What's Not "Already" Yours

Stress comes from either desiring something you already have, as mentioned earlier, or desiring something you can't have. Let's say you see, in a shop window, a beautiful gold watch. You desire to own it *but* can't afford it right now. Just as the "but" splits the sentence in two, it also splits the mind in two. If you could afford that watch, you wouldn't *desire* it; you'd simply buy it! You'd see it, like it and buy it. There are no "buts" about it. No desire, conflict or stress is involved. The secret of contentment, then, is this: if you can have a thing, have it, but if you can't – don't desire it. In other words, don't desire what's not *already* yours.

On the subconscious level you're already at your goal weight or behavior, so desiring it would backfire or short circuit your realizing that goal. It's like the first rule of closing a sale: When the prospect finally says yes to the salesperson's offer, the salesperson should immediately stop talking, because anything uttered thereafter would do nothing but jeopardize the sale. Mentally and emotionally you have already lost that weight, so stop desiring it. Only in this state of desirelessness can the weight-loss sale be consummated.

You can, however, *create* what is not yours. If you would have the watch you want or the body you want, then make it a creative activity instead of an emotional one. To desire is emotional – of a lower faculty; to create is spiritual. Longing for anything is incompatible with reality because, consciously or unconsciously, your organism already knows what your needs and desires are and is already working toward their attainment.

Whether or not you're aware of it, you're always heading in the direction of total fulfillment. The key is to just be more aware of your intention and more receptive to receiving it. All things being equal, your goal weight is already yours; it's already programmed into your genes. The whole task of detached intelligence is to just keep "all things equal," to just get out of the way and let nature run its course, to just follow the leading of common sense, and to not ignore it when stress reminds you that you've gone astray. You are, and have always been, the only hindrance to success. If you want to know what's the problem, just look in the mirror. By desiring, you effectively contradict your own self, your own organism. It's like turning on the car's starter while the engine is already running, or driving with the emergency brake on. How frustrating and self-defeating. When tired, sleep; when hungry, eat. When sated, stop eating. No desiring, dieting or willpower is involved.

The Law of Reverse Effort

According to Newton's Law, "All action produces an equal and opposite reaction." If you emotionally want to lose weight, you'll gain more weight – as you've likely experienced. Emotional activity brings about the opposite of what we want by the same principle that propels a rocket or a jet airplane. In a balanced universe, movement one way *must* be compensated for by an equivalent movement the opposite way in order to maintain the balance. The plane's propulsion in one direction, propels the plane toward the opposite direction. So to make the plane go east, we aim the energy west. If we want the rocket to go up, we aim the energy down. And in the same way, if we want pain, we exert energy toward pleasure and gratification.

But we can't apply this principle in reverse as the masochist attempts to do. We can't say, "I will then seek pleasure through pain." This doesn't work either, for seeking pain is just as ineffectual – long term, as seeking pleasure. Again, the problem is not *what* you emotionally seek but *that* you emotionally seek.

The universe turns in only one direction and that direction is *neutral.* If happiness and weight loss is your intention, then neutrality (being centered) is the direction you'd have to travel to get there. Think of a revolving door as the world. The door panel in front of you is "pleasure" – the pleasure of being your goal weight. The door behind you is "pain"– the pain of being overweight. When you push toward pleasure, pain comes right on your heels.

Now let's say the revolving doors are in motion. Perhaps there's someone in the compartment in front of you and someone in the one behind you. They're doing all the pushing. All you have to do now is to just go along for the ride. You don't have to push for pleasure but just remain neutrally centered by moving at the same speed the doors (the world) are moving.

This is a good example of creative movement where you are still and in action at the same time. You are moving but are still with respect to the doors. As far as the doors are concerned, you are not moving at all. The world is moving and you are moving with it. You're in unison. You and the world are not in stressful conflict, not moving in different directions or at different speeds but are equal in all respects.

A *Seesaw Named Desire*

Think of the world as a child's seesaw. One end is "pleasure," the other is "pain," and you – the higher you, are situated at the center. The seesaw is in perfect balance; that is, until you begin to step out in the direction of "pleasure" causing it to fall and "pain" to simultaneously rise up to become dominant.

Desiring is like trying to remove a speck from your soup. As you approach the speck with your spoon, it slips away, and the quicker you chase it, the quicker it moves away. The only way to catch it is to chase it creatively rather than emotionally. Instead of *moving* after it, be *still* and let it come to you. Be receptive – by lowering the spoon to just below the surface (the subconscious) of the soup, so the speck flows into the spoon naturally, by gravity. Thus, you attain it without chasing it. The speck wasn't the problem; the approach was the problem.

The reason the speck eludes the spoon so naturally is because they are physically connected so have no choice. The soup is the medium connecting spoon and speck. It's the physical link that also separates them. Just as a car and its trailer stay separate by virtue of the hitch between them, so the spoon and the speck stay separate by virtue of the soup between them.

The way it works physically is the way it works emotionally: Pain and pleasure are directly linked but we don't notice the connection because it's so subtle in the same way that we don't notice the soup as a connective because it's so un-solid or unsubstantial. Thus pain and pleasure are connected as two sides of one continuous mind. They're a continuum. If you emote toward pleasure you come to pain; if you try to escape, it follows like a shadow.

Your only alternative is to transcend the whole coin. Rise above it by living on the center rim of the coin instead of on either surface of it. By remaining at the center, the point and attitude of detached indifference, you experience natural pleasure *all* of the time instead of emotional (false) pleasure *some* of the time. Your appetite comes and remains under effortless control. Pounds drop in due course.

Attachment To Pleasure Changes It To Pain

If you're experiencing pleasure while eating and try to prolong that pleasure by eating beyond satiety – you quickly lose the pleasure. Just as emotional effort toward pleasure causes pain, so does trying to hang onto the pleasure you're experiencing also causes pain. Clinging to anything is, in effect, an attempt to deny what is. A person finding a slice of chocolate cake delicious and gratifying would like to prolong that pleasure, so she has another slice. But the second slice is not quite as good as the first, and the third is about to make her ill. What was delicious a few slices ago has become a virtual toxin. Clinging attachment caused what was sweet to turn sour, not because the *cake* had changed each time, but because the *situation* had changed each time. Attachment rather than detachment caused what was beautiful to quickly become ugly.

Indifference To Pleasure Causes It To Remain

If you can experience the *sensual* pleasure of food without being emotionally affected by it, then there will simply be no need or desire to overeat. When you don't get excited about anything, especially food, you are then simply being yourself – happy and content. When you're content, your mind is still like a placid lake; when excited, it ripples in agitation. It was relaxed and centered, but your emotional response disturbed it, affected it. So by remaining unmoved or unchanged by the beauty, smell and taste of the food, the sensual pleasure doesn't change either. You eat when the body is hungry and stop when the hunger subsides. Happiness and appetite-control are enjoying food without getting anything out of it but physical nourishment and sensual pleasure. And that's all you need.

Trying To Escape Pain Causes It To Persist

Running from discomfort doesn't work for the same reason chasing gratification doesn't work – they're both emotional activities and anything emotional must, by law, backfire.

They are, in effect, equally negative. In desire we get the opposite of what we want; in escape we get more of what we're trying to escape from. This principle can be seen in the same revolving door illustration used earlier. There we saw that in pushing the pleasure of food, we caused pain to come upon us. Here, by pushing to escape the pain-door – it follows us like a shadow. The actions in both cases are the same, only the motives are different. And both are doomed to failure, again, not because their motives are right or wrong but because both are emotional rather than creative.

Whatever we try to escape, avoid, resist or suppress – we endow with power. Emotional discomfort, in and of itself, has no power to harm us; it is merely a signaling device, an indicator, a messenger. By avoiding the messenger we, in effect, make the messenger the issue instead of the imbalance it represents. The messenger then mistakenly becomes the evil with which we have to deal. It becomes what we must escape, resist, struggle with or kill. It's what we must drown with alcohol, kill with drugs, engorge with food, distract with excitement, etc. But this error is insidious and insatiable. A bottomless pit.

The Creative Versus The Emotional

When you attempt to treat the symptom rather than the cause, nothing works. The ego is stubborn and foolish. It refuses to see and admit its error, refuses to see that its self-centered perspective is a false one. So it spends its life in denial, trying to avoid the truth or trying to prove a lie is the truth. Here you can see the need for rigorous self-honesty and self-awareness if you are to lose weight.

In this we see the basic difference between the creative and the emotional: The creative lives in truth; the emotional lives in a lie or in fantasy. The creative is at peace; the emotional is disturbed. The creative comes from contentment; the emotional comes from hunger.

Accepting Pain Changes it to Pleasure

When you allow and accept the pain you're experiencing, that pain naturally converts to pleasure. The most effective remedy for handling emotional discomfort is simply to experience it fully and indifferently. To the degree discomfort is allowed rather than rejected, it disappears. The positive attitude of acceptance cancels or neutralizes the negative discomfort. It balances it out of existence. It transcends it, corrects it.

Emotional agitation is relaxed simply by virtue of the still, passive, detached awareness of the agitation. The agitation relaxes by itself. When you're experiencing discomfort without "desiring" that it should leave or without attempting to escape it (escapism), you're then in a state of centered indifference in which discomfort cannot exist. And if discomfort doesn't exist, neither does the desire to overeat.

Emotional discomfort becomes obsolete simply through the indifferent allowance and acceptance of it. In other words, to eliminate anything negative or unpleasant we move *into* it not away from it. We confront it rather than resist it. Pain and pleasure are a single continuum like the inside of the cup that continues to the outside of the cup. By entering the pain we eventually come to the pleasure, just as by entering far enough into the night the day must appear. As night becomes day, so does pain become pleasure. If feeling depressed, for instance, you'd do nothing about it except witness it indifferently. You wouldn't like it, hate it, want it to stay or want it to leave, but would indifferently observe it out of existence.

The word *pain* comes from the Greek and Latin meaning *penalty*. Pain is the penalty we pay for violating the Law of Detachment. Whenever there's discomfort, whether from boredom, guilt, worry, resentment, anxiousness, depression, self-doubt, fear, uncertainty, etc., just allow it. Think of it as just a temporary aberration. Don't interfere with it in any way. The negativity came from emotional involvement in the first place. To reverse the process, we don't want to feed it more of the same. To reverse the process, our relationship with negativity of any name or nature, has to be one of detachment from it, not one of entanglement or engrossment in it.

Appreciating Your Pain

You allow and accept your discomfort knowing that its sole purpose is to lead you back to the truth that would free you from it. To appreciate a thing is to totally experience it. Any discomfort experienced to the end must leave you. There's simply no place for pain to gain a foothold. Whenever tension arises, don't be averse to it but enter into it. Relish it as an opportunity to regain more or your lost joy, freedom and control. Look it straight in the eye with calm, firm indifference and watch it vaporize out of existence. Passive, creative energy works like a light that makes the dark disappear. As darkness is merely the absence of light, so pain is merely the absence of objective awareness. By shining impartial attention on pain or craving, you expose its nothingness, its superficialness. The two can't exist simultaneously.

Contentment is the total acceptance of people, places and things just as they are. We have to relate to everything if we are to relate to anything. And likewise, we have to accept ourselves in our totality as well. We're just as complex as the world is, the product of countless generations – and perhaps lives, of evolutionary development. Everything we ever were is within us now, and everything we'll ever become is also within us now. We consist of so many conflicting thoughts, feelings, attitudes and beliefs, that the only way to relate to them all is to indifferently accept them all. Otherwise, we'd become insane or neurotic – like a centipede trying to figure out which leg to use next.

You don't have to understand all things at all times. If you are feeling jealousy, sadness, resentment, hate, greed, loneliness, boredom, cravings, etc., allow it. Accept it. At those moments, that's what you are. To deny with guilt, regret or shame is disordered thinking that leads to disordered eating.

Any discomfort you repress or suppress becomes a toxin that will taint your whole being. It will negatively color all that you say, think, feel and do. Emotional eating means something is eating you. Think of negativity as a mental or emotional bacteria that eats you to the degree you are attached to it. Attachment gives it a septic home or foundation from which to fester into fat or disease. When you are detachedly aware of your anger, the anger is controlled – period. It's like the effect of "counting to ten." It subsides. It *must* subside. "Keeping your distance" is the controlling factor. Anger is a neutral energy, but becomes explosive when repressed. When anger or resentment is thus controlled, your appetite becomes controlled – nullifying the desire to eat beyond satiety.

Remember the distinction that negative feelings are *what* you are, not *who* you are. Who you are is the pure, detached awareness that's above it all – above all inner and outer experience.

Creating Your Own Conflicts

If you emotionally desire, try, wish, hope to control your appetite, then you'll fail. It cannot be otherwise for again, they are two sides of the same mind. If you would be happy and successful at this, then be so. Why bring desire or effort into the picture? By desiring you introduce a conflict into the equation that doesn't exist. You make struggle a foregone conclusion before even beginning. You create resistance by anticipating it. *To fight something is to feed it.* That's the meaning of the saying, "Resist not evil." You create an adversary relationship between you and your goal that's fictitious. Your goal doesn't care if it's attained by you or not. It's totally indifferent to your designs upon it. It's just sitting there to be or not be partaken of. By desiring, you place it on a pedestal and give it artificial prominence. The more emotional the desire the greater the prominence. You set yourself up to fail by creating blocks where none exist. For every desire there *must* also be a complementary block built into it. Where there's no block there's no desire, and where no desire, no block.

In reality you can't desire and you can't try; you either have it or you don't. The only question to ask yourself, then, is whether you have it. If not, no amount of desire and effort will help. A flower doesn't desire or use effort to grow; it simply grows. It has a direction but not a desire. A desire is emotional and failure prone, while direction is creative and success prone.

The flower's "goal" is pre-determined and inherent, so doesn't need to desire. It's virtually already where it's going. It's just a matter of time. The purpose of a flower is to bloom to its full potential. And its source of power is the sun. Now all it has to do is let go and be itself in the direction of its source – and creation happens of its own accord. "Spring comes and the grass grows by itself," is the Zen saying. No emotional desire, effort or ego ambition is involved. It's just being itself, and to just be is to spontaneously flower. It just relaxes, and out of that stillness, out of that "holy indifference" it joyously blooms into the richest colors and sweetest perfumes. So the pounds drop by themselves.

"Perhaps everything we believe is false."
−Descartes

Living in reality is understanding that, to some degree or other, you're indeed personally biased with respect to practically all that you think, feel and do, and as a result, lose some degree of clarity and power. It's not a question of maybe we're biased or to what degree, but that we are. Being present in the flesh, in and of itself, implies the existence of a self-centered bias. The point is that we don't *have* a bias, we *are* a bias. The eyes can't see themselves because the eyes are the things doing the seeing. The nose can't smell itself for the same reason, and so on with all the senses. And likewise with thoughts and feelings. Thoughts can't think of themselves and feelings can't feel themselves. That's the blind spot of clarity and power. That's the existential handicap we have to overcome. We overcome it by getting *outside* of ourselves, getting *above* ourselves. We have to be on the outside looking in as well as on the inside looking out. That's what detachment is, and that's how you get above an eating disorder and all the stress and negative feelings that trigger and trail it.

Think of yourself as a business organization with your thoughts, feelings and five senses serving as your seven key employees, and you are the objective overseer. The thinking faculty does all the planning and organizing for you. It's the brains of the organization, the computer. The body is your eyes and ears, and also does all the legwork for you. The feelings inform you whether things are going as planned. And you, the higher awareness, remain above them all, and by virtue of your aboveness, you control them all.

The way the employer maintains control is by keeping an appropriate distance from his employees so that their respective roles don't conflict. You allow them to play their roles without influencing or affecting their report; and likewise, you don't allow their report to personally (emotionally) influence or affect you. In this way, the parts work together for the good of the whole. They are independent and in harmony at the same time. Everything's under natural and effortless control. When your mind is so organized and ordered, so will be your appetite.

Controlling The Mind

Mind control is nothing more than watching its activity from an appropriate distance. By observing thoughts, feelings and sensations as if they were outside of you – which they really are, you control those activities. Nothing else has to be done. Detached awareness, in and of itself, is the controlling factor. You are not desiring to stop, repress or change the mind by force, but just to witness it as it is. By simply witnessing it, you control or change it.

Mind-body activity is like a child at play. To control him, we don't have to bridle him; we just watch him. To watch is to control. He can't begin to get into mischief because we're right there, right on top of the situation – above it all. The same with the mind: negative or misleading thoughts or feelings can't begin to harm you because you're there at the moment of their inception. By observing mind-body activities from a distance, it becomes obvious that they, in and of themselves, have absolutely no power over you. You needn't be controlled by either negative or positive feelings. As far as your higher awareness is concerned, they are *just* feelings. That's what being relaxed, centered and free is, and that's what your true nature is.

Higher Self-Consciousness

Socrates condensed all wisdom into two words: *"Know Thyself."* If you know how your mind-body works, it's much easier to control yourself. If you don't know how you tick, you just repeat the same error indefinitely. By witnessing thoughts, feelings and behavior from a distance, you're able to see *first hand* who you are and why you eat as you do.

To the degree you can – and you'll get better with practice, notice all mental activity. Just pay attention to it, as it is, whenever it occurs. Know that you're thinking whenever you're thinking. When thinking about going to a restaurant, *know* that's what you're thinking. When playing tennis and thinking you might win or lose, witness yourself thinking those thoughts. When reflecting on a problem at work, watch yourself thinking the matter over and deciding on a course of action. When you find yourself daydreaming or musing, catch yourself doing it.

Are you thinking of what you'll wear, what you'll say, what might be the response to what you say? Thinking of hurting someone, helping someone? Thinking about money, food, sex, reading, writing, retirement? Be detachedly aware that you are. And even when there's no thought activity at all, be conscious of that too. By persistently and choicelessly witnessing your thoughts and feelings in this way, you'll soon break the false identity or attachment you have with those thoughts and so regain control in the process. It will become clear that you're indeed above and in control of your thoughts. Once you know you can control your thoughts, you'll know that you can control your whole life. This is not about being *personally* self-conscious; it's about being *higher* self-conscious.

Increasing Emotional Awareness

Your attitude with respect to all feeling is that they're all alike; they're all the same to you. One feeling is just as good or bad or right or wrong as any other. You don't feel guilty about the one, nor saintly about the other. From the perspective of an impersonal, impartial observer, there's no difference between a negative feeling and a positive feeling; they're both just feelings. In other words, "No matter how you slice it, it's still baloney." The rule of thumb is this: If it's a mental activity, no matter how lowly or noble, it's not real but a concept or an illusion. It may or not become real later, but at this stage, it's just imagination. And it's just this detachment that'll give you the power to wisely discriminate between which thoughts you'll discard, and which you'll convert to actuality.

You control feelings the same way you control thought, by observing them from a distance. By witnessing your feelings without letting them get under your skin, you effectively correct the wrong relationship you've been having with them. You put emotion back in its proper place – as the employee not the employer, as the subordinate not the superior. Feelings are to inform not to control. When a feeling arises for or against something, whether negative, positive, painful or pleasurable, do not react to it in any way, but just witness it with calm disinterest.

If some person, place or thing is irritating you, just observe the fact of that irritation and nothing else. You're not concerned with whether the irritation is justified – you're not a judge; you're only concerned with the fact that it *exists*. If irritation is what you're feeling in that moment, just acknowledge, admit and accept it. Also acknowledge that it's not *you* that's irritated; it's the *feelings* that are irritated. The "you" are above them. See the difference? Then, by virtue of the laws of allowance and detachment, the negative ones will leave, and the positive ones will remain.

If you can stand back and witness the irritation from a distance, you'll see that the irritation originated with you, personally. It was of your doing, your responsibility. You did it to yourself by owning or identifying with the feeling. You made the feeling who and what you are. Your feelings have taken you over, and an outside agency is pulling the strings or pressing the buttons. Instead of observing the situation from a distance, you became   personally, emotionally, egotistically involved. You violated the integrity of whatever role you happened to be playing at the time. You took a social, business or family situation and personalized it.

If a person acts improperly, it's not your emotional (personal) business; it's the business of your *role* to respond accordingly. If you were a judge and were provoked by a lawyer, you'd hold him in "contempt." The contempt the judge "feels" is not personal but official. In the same way, if your child's behavior is "out of order," the matter would be handled parentally not personally. The same applies in any relationship. The offended party would not react personally, but in a manner appropriate to the role and situation. More on this in the next chapter, *Taking Life Impersonally*.

Living In Indifference Is Living In Reality

Reality isn't concerned whether you're sad or happy, bored or excited, guilty or innocent, doubtful or confident, angry or forgiving. As far as reality is concerned, they're all the same; they're just feelings. Carl Sagan said, "The universe seems neither benign nor hostile, merely indifferent."

Reality is like an empty cup – totally indifferent to what's poured into it. It doesn't accept one beverage over another, but is equally receptive to and unaffected by whatever's poured into it. Similarly, a flashlight doesn't shine more on some things than others; it shines equally on everything. And a flashlight doesn't change according to what it shines on either. Both the beautiful and the ugly have no affect on it. It remains true to itself – just an impartial, detached flashlight. If we can remain in reality by adopting the attitude of the cup or the flashlight, all fear and conflict would be eliminated, and along with it, the false need or desire to overeat.

Fear is always of the unknown, and conflict is always of one feeling or thought against its opposite. If you understand that life consists of nothing but negative and positive thoughts and feelings, then you know all there is to know.

And if you know that the negative and positive are exactly alike, as far as your higher consciousness is concerned, then there can be no conflict. You know all there is to know, and know how to respond to it. There's nothing else. You've got it. Now you're free. Now you're really enlightened, educated and cultivated – no longer ignorant. You know universal convention and can move within it with freedom, ease and confidence. Now you can relax and enjoy life and food without getting carried away by either.

Whatever comes into your cup, whether pleasant or unpleasant, embrace it without judgment. Don't wrestle with it, argue with it, or entertain it in any way. Do not love it, hate it or fear it. Don't accept or reject it; but just be indifferently aware of it. You're playing the role of a cup and the appropriate behavior for a cup is to not get attached to the contents. Don't allow your contents to push or pull you or raise or lower you; but remain firmly in the center of them. Neither indulge nor repress them – just witness them from a distance.

When you thus break the identification with your contents (your lower faculties), you're no longer subject to them; they become subject to you. You're no longer subject to the world; the world (your body) becomes subject to you, so you can stop overeating at will.

Key Points and Principles:

1. That stress is the primary trigger and fuel for overeating.

2. That you control stress by keeping an appropriate and respectable distance from all that you see, hear, think, feel and do.

3. That the *emotional* pursuit of pleasure causes stress.

4. That trying to cling to pleasure causes stress.

5. That indifference to pleasure causes it to remain.

6. That trying to escape from stress causes it to remain.

7. That accepting stress changes it to relaxation or serenity.

8. That the real you are above thought, feeling and food.

9. That detachment breaks the vicious circle where: emotional desire causes stress; stress blocks clarity; lack of clarity causes error; error causes failure, failure causes stress all over again.

CHAPTER 9
TAKING LIFE IMPERSONALLY

"All the world's a stage and all the men and women, merely players." – Shakespeare

If you're going to be an impersonal, non-emotional eater, then you'll have to be an impersonal, non-emotional person as well. If a particular method gives you clarity and power at the dinner table, it will also give you clarity and power everywhere and all the time. This is what makes the Method universal.

The "How to Act" Principle

Shakespeare's statement is not just clever metaphor; it's literal truth. The *law of detachment* applies not only to being above all that you think, feel and eat; it also applies to being above all the roles you play – for the same reason: Being above and distinct from the roles you play is the way to control yourself and your behavior. It's living in reality. Just as your thoughts, feelings and senses are not *really* you, so the roles you play are not *really* you. They're just acts you perform to suit the occasion. The real you are consciously above them all.

Here again, to know yourself is to control yourself and your appetite. This "truth" of what you really are is the controlling factor. Understanding the distinction between who you are and how to act resolves the conflict that diminishes power over your life.

When you know yourself in this sense, you know virtually everything. Nothing else needs to be done but to practice keeping a respectable distance from the personal roles you play – including the role of yourself as a consciously detached eater. When you see eating as just another "role" to be played, you tend to play it more mindfully and meaningfully. It becomes a meditation. You're on the outside looking in at your eating instead of being mindlessly mired in it.

The "Situation is Everything" Principle

How does one "act" in an emotionally-controlled, conflict-free way? The answer is by *letting the situation determine your role, and letting the role determine your behavior.* The "situation" is the relationship in which you find yourself at any given moment, and your "role" is the particular part you play in that relationship, such as employer/employee, clerk/customer, husband/wife, parent/child, professional /client, etc., and correct behavior is that which is *appropriate* to that role.

Thus you act, but not according to your personal bias or ego; you act according to a role determined by the *situation. Your ego has been effectively detached from the decision-making process.* There's no longer a conflict of personality. You now act according to the fact of the situation rather than the biased opinion of the personality. You act according to principle rather than caprice.

To the degree you do, you live confidently instead of insecurely. Calmly instead of tensely. You become more free-flowing, more actual, more yourself. You move from role-to-role with the ease and grace of a ballerina rather than the fearful studiedness of an automaton. And the beauty of it is, you don't have to think about it; it's all unpremeditated, all unstressful. Freedom means decisions are simpler, less complicated. You become more decisive. And all you have to do is know the situation you're in, know your role in it, then *act* accordingly to the best of your ability.

Keeping Your Distance

All parties in a relationship have a certain role that determines how each is expected to behave. In order for society to function in an orderly and efficient way, it's members must act in conformance with certain conventions of behavior. The clerk is expected to behave in a certain way with respect to his customer, and the customer, with respect to the clerk. And likewise in the relationships between professional and client, teacher and student, parent and offspring, husband and wife, employer and employee, etc. Each has an obligation and responsibility to act towards the other in a manner characteristic of the role being played.

Being in Relationship

As our subject is "acting," it'll be useful to think in theatrical or literary terms. Think of yourself as the main character in a play. You, the protagonist, are the person around whom the play or story revolves. You're the center of the action, the center of attraction. But you're not there alone, not there in a vacuum; you're there and you act in relationship with the persons and things in the scene with you. You are never really alone, never really not in relationship with someone or something. In one scene you're at home with your family and playing the role of "husband" or "wife" with respect to your spouse, or "mother" or "father" with respect to your children. In another scene, you're at work playing the part of a "co-worker" with respect to other co-workers, or the alternating roles of "manager" to your subordinates and "subordinate" to your managers. In other scenes, you are playing the role of a "spectator" at a performance, "participant" at a social gathering, "friend" with respect to a friend, and so on.

Even when alone you're playing a role such as a "listener" with respect to music, a "viewer" with respect to television, a "reader" with respect to your newspaper, a "diner" with respect to eating, etc. These scenes are the ever-changing backgrounds, settings and contexts in which you, the central character, perform.

In all these scenes, you're there in relation or connection to someone or something else. Even when alone, you are relating to yourself, to your higher self's consciousness or to your lower self's thoughts, feelings and desires. In a universe where all things are connected, it's impossible *not* to be related to something at any given moment. The key to good acting is always knowing what is that person, place or thing. If you don't know how your presence is immediately pertinent to a situation, you can't know what your proper role is or how to play it correctly. You won't know how to act. You'll feel insecure about your acting ability. Clarity and power over yourself, therefore, come from thinking of all situations in terms of *relationships*. So when you're eating, you're in a relationship with food – with you the controller, and food the controlled.

Same Actor, Different Roles

Once reality is understood as a relationship, it becomes obvious that the role you play in it is also "real" – not *absolutely* real, but real in the sense that it's compatible and consistent with how to function in the world, how to function in harmony with the world so as to be in "control" of it. Roles are not you in the higher spiritual sense; they're you in the lower, personal sense. In the spiritual sense your "identity" never changes; you are always the impersonal observer *above* everything including all the roles you play. On the personal level, your identity must constantly change to accord with the situation or circumstance. Thus, by "playing a role" you *are* being real; you are being in tune with reality. To not play a role is to live in error and powerlessness.

Put another way, your role is not *who* you are; it's what you do. It's your work, duty, function, position, or office. A "judge" is not *really* a judge but just *acts* a judge when "on the bench." When he leaves the courthouse, he no longer acts as judge but as "husband" to his wife, "father" to his children, etc. And likewise, "parents" are not *really* parents in the higher sense, but just play the role of parents. That a role comes by way of a biological relationship rather than a social or business one doesn't make it any less a role to be detachedly played.

Reality doesn't differentiate between biology and society. All roles, regardless of their level or genesis, must be played in the orderly and principled manner appropriate to them. To the degree they are, there's harmony and control; to the degree they're not, there's conflict. The conflict comes from the false identity of confusing who you are with what you do. You are both a human being and a human doing. Being is who you really are; doing is just an act, just a transient part you play.

You Are Not Really Napolean

The difference is one of perspective. Before, you didn't think in terms of "playing a role" because you were so self-centeredly identified with everything you did, that you believed you actually *were* all the parts you played. You couldn't separate the actor from the act – which is a form of insanity, like the actor who convinced himself that he really is Napoleon. So the difference between conscious and unconscious role-playing is that in the one case, you emotionally identify with your role – you think it's really you; and in the other case, you see yourself as separate from it, above it, detached from it. You see your role merely as a human convention, just a "hat" to be worn; not as something to take personally, but as something to be taken creatively or recreationally.

The role itself is artificial but your act is real. You are the artist, and your role is your medium. Playing a role doesn't mean you are not yourself; on the contrary, you are fully yourself, but *you are yourself in the context of your role.* The role provides the necessary vehicle or means by which you *can* express yourself authentically. To be authentic simply means to be uniquely yourself. And since you already are yourself – and cannot be anything other no matter how much you try, all that remains is to have some vehicle or platform from which to express. Your family, social, business and professional roles provide that platform. If you are playing the role of a waiter, business person, housekeeper, artist, doctor, clerk, parent – it's your own unique personality that distinguishes you from all others playing the same role. Your role, like the body in which you live, is superficial, but the personality that animates and gives it expression, is authentic – and that's the source of your personal power.

The Real Actor Can Play Any Role

The mark of an authentic actor is his adaptability. He can move with equal ease into any role, while the bad or false actor is limited in the types of roles he can play. The false actor is like a painter who can paint landscapes but not seascapes, or like a novelist who can write mysteries but not romances, or like a salesperson who can sell oranges but not apples. These are not real artists. A real painter can paint anything, a real writer can write anything, a real salesperson can sell anything. In whatever situation you find yourself, what matters is that you're real, and being consciously an actor is *how* to be real, is the *method* of being real. Where there's no personality disorder there's no eating disorder.

The authentic actor has the flexibility of a chameleon – whose color is not fixed, but changes with his environment. When on a brown tree, he turns brown; when on a green leaf he becomes green. If you asked him what color he is, he could only say, "It depends on the situation." Or, if he was a sales chameleon, he might say, "What color do you want?" Similarly, when the authentic actor is in Rome, he dances the Tarantella; when in Tel Aviv, he sings *Havah Nagilah*. If he's poor, he does without; if rich, he lives lavishly. When at a wedding banquet, he plays the "celebrant"; at a funeral, he becomes a "mourner." *Knowing how to act is knowing how to live.*

If the chameleon didn't change colors he'd stand out, exposing himself to danger. Likewise, if a person was cheerful at a funeral and somber at a wedding, he too would stand out and be in danger – of being shunned by his fellows. He would not be in harmony with the situation, not be "one" with it. We say such a person doesn't know how to act, doesn't know his part. He's an outcast, isolated from the situation rather than related to it. This isolation makes him a stranger instead of a participant. He may not like the situation he's in, but that's beside the point. As an actor, that's none of his business. The point of fact is, he's there, so is obliged to act accordingly. Likes and dislikes are personal, emotional considerations – not part of the real actor's persona. They are irrelevant to the reality of the situation and one's role in it. The real actor is only concerned with what is, and that his response is *equal* to it.

The Service Principle

The authentic actor doesn't have a "self" from which to like or dislike. He has no passions, feelings or desires of his own ego. He's just an actor, just a selfless medium. Whatever he feels is not for himself, but for his role. He feels with the situation or person he's with. If you're hurt, he's hurt; if you're happy, he's happy. Whatever you want is what he wants; wherever you want to go is where he wants to go. His being is virtually determined by you. You're the director of the play. For of himself he is already fulfilled, already "there," so has no need to do anything else but to give or serve.

So this serving is more than just a "good" thing, it's a *law* based on the fact that when you're above it all, there's nothing left to do but give. A servant is what you are and what you do. It's your *modus operandi,* your underlying motive in all relationship – personal and business.

Conscious and constant service to others is the love/wisdom-based method of transforming from self-centeredness to other-centeredness. Service is the natural method or "technique" for getting out of yourself, for expressing yourself. You are a "method" actor, and service is your secret, all powerful method of expression.

This explains why we feel good when we donate to charity or help a person or animal in need. Even the simplest thing like giving directions to a lost driver makes us feel good. Why? Because *serving is the fulfillment of our purpose in life.* It's the essential expression of the selfless, egoless soul.

Validating Others

Service is regarding and appreciating others. A basic human need is to be appreciated for who we are. We're all special in that there's no one in the world quite like us. While being different is nothing of which to be "proud"; it is something to be recognized. People *are* different. Relating to them, therefore, implies relating to their differences. If we are to connect to a person at all, we must recognize, understand and regard that person. There's no other way. To be with someone and not appreciate his uniqueness is to not *really* be with him except on the most superficial and meaningless level.

Appreciating and recognizing the specialness of others is correct and good, and we certainly *will* benefit from it – for giving is the way of getting, but that's not why we do it. We do it because it's essential to authentic relationship and the fulfillment of being.

We respect a person by being sensitively aware of his presence. Awareness and sensitivity require energy, and merely applying energy to a person, in and of itself, is being respectful and validating. It's to listen with undivided attention – not with your mind elsewhere, or casting judgment, or listening with an ear to how this person may be useful to you. You're listening for the purpose of understanding that person, understanding how *you* can be of use to that person – nothing else. The authentic actor lives in a service-based relationship with others, while the false actor lives in a self-centered one – then overeats to relieve the resulting boredom, loneliness, lack of intimacy and general failure of the relationship.

Of course, this *principle of service* applies commercially and professionally as well personally. To the degree you think of benefiting the client/customer first rather than yourself first, you'll be far more effective in "selling" yourself and your product, service or idea.

The Integrity of The Relationship

All roles are "professional" in that they are played, not according to personal feelings, but to the dictates of the role itself. And as there's never a time when you're not playing some role (except when sleeping), there's never a time when you act according to uncontrolled feelings.

Keeping a respectable distance between one another's role means we respect the sanctity of both the individual and the role he's playing. We respect the inviolable privacy of the individual. We don't get too familiar with anyone and don't allow anyone to get too familiar with us. "Familiarity breeds contempt" because it violates privacy and the integrity of the relationship. To have our privacy or "space" invaded is to have our soul or center taken over so that we're no longer our own secure selves but are now being used or exploited.

The same principle applies to food. We keep an emotional distance from food so as not to violate the integrity of the relationship – and overeat as a consequence. The role of the eater is, again, to eat for physical purposes not emotional purposes.

Key Points and Principles:

1. That knowing yourself is key to controlling yourself.

2. That to know yourself is to know your role in every situation.

3. That there's no time or place when you're not playing a role.

4. That you're above and distinct from every role you play.

5. That you act according to role not to feelings.

6. That you allow the situation to determine your role, and your role to determine your behavior.

7. That service to others, personal, business or professional, is the principle and purpose of all human behavior and relationship.

CHAPTER 10
SEIZING THE MOMENT

"The past and future are imaginary." – WFM

Neither the past nor the future are "real," so neither has the power to change your mind or body. The present moment is the point of the six C's: calmness, contentment, centeredness, clarity, control and confidence. Only here-now now can the mind be relaxed, satisfied and super aware. Being present means total involvement in, and knowledge of, what you're thinking, feeling and eating. It means your attention isn't conflicted or scattered.

When eating, showering, dressing or driving, for instance, notice that your mind is only partially there. And if you trace your activities through the day, you'll see that the mind is seldom on the thing at hand – especially eating. This is the uncentered, uncontrolled, overweight mindset.

We think we're more productive when "multi-tasking," for example, but the reverse is true: Not focusing on one thing at a time, in the present, makes us less productive and intelligent because the energy of awareness is dissipated and diffused. We're scatterbrained. We don't really know what a shower feels like. Don't really know what food tastes like. We don't remember people's names, what we just read, etc. We're like a person in a day-dream or trance who misses his exit on the highway, or like a drunk in a blackout who makes it home, but doesn't have a clue how he did it. The idea that the mundane is not worthy of awareness is to miss the point that the present is the point of clarity and appetite-control power regardless of the object.

If you're not present in the shower, you won't be very present while eating either. Your awareness has become lethargic or atrophied. Being present is not only a discipline, it's the mother of all disciplines, for if you're not all here, you're not all there. The saying "Use it or lose it" applies to the higher faculty of awareness as it does to thinking, feeling, and the five senses. In fact, it applies especially to the higher, for the higher consciousness is your *central guidance or reference point* by which you control all the lower faculties.

Remember that any mind-body transformation can only occur in the present moment: Only in the here-now can you be detachedly conscious, maintain your new self-image, control your appetite, exercise your body and neutralize your stress.

Overcoming Temptation

To be effective and secure, one doesn't have to refer to the past or look to the future, for both are inherent in the present and stored in your subconscious mind. The present is a self-contained universe that doesn't require anything external to it. Anything from the past that would be useful and relevant to this moment will spontaneously spring up from the subconscious and be available to you. It's always at hand. You don't have to "remember" that all actions have consequences; you just have to be alert in the present moment. When alert, all ramifications and resolutions present themselves simultaneously. Before you eat beyond satiety, for example, you won't have to "think it through," for you'll know very well the ramifications of such a mindless act because – via present-moment detachment, you are no longer mindless, no longer in a trance, so to speak.

Temptation is no longer a factor. You transcend it. It's a low and obsolete emotion that you've gone beyond. Yes, you'll still feel temptation on occasion because it's been part of your mindset your whole life. It's part of the human condition. The point is that now you don't have to *act* on it. You have the power of choice now. Just because you *feel* like eating the wrong food at the wrong time, doesn't mean you have to. It's okay to *think* of shooting someone, but you wouldn't actually do it. Momentary discomfort is not the end of world. It always passes, and you feel so much better about yourself for not succumbing. Success builds on success. Confidence builds on confidence.

Present-moment detachment increases your emotional intelligence. If you're in the past – *remembering* the "comfort" you got from food, or if you're in the future – *anticipating* the "comfort" that a gratuitous extra helping might bring you – then you'll succumb. In the present moment, right and wrong present themselves at the same time, so the choice becomes clear. The way to go becomes obvious. It's not complicated; it's just about doing what you know is right, and if you're present, you'll have the power to do so.

The Present is the Point of Security

If a person is alert in the present, the future will provide for itself; if not, nothing from the past will help. By living from the past, he'll either repeat the same mistakes over and over, or make different ones all the time. He'll find himself always "chalking things up to experience," doing and saying the wrong thing at the wrong time, not being quite "with it." Always being "a day late and a dollar short." Reality is happening, but he'll be constantly out of sync with it, constantly lagging a bit behind because he must always refer to his memory before responding. Even if it's for just a split-second, it's too late. The moment has passed. The boat has been missed. He overeats. Life's happening *now* and must be responded to *now*. To miss by only a hair is still to miss. To eat just an ounce beyond satiety will keep you overweight.

The ordinary person erroneously "believes" that by leaving his comfort zone of the past, he'd be as if lost in space, without any point of reference. He needs something to hang onto, some kind of tether or security blanket – which in this case is food.

So the person not fully present lives in a false sense of security. False because he's no more secure than an ostrich hiding its head in the sand. Responding to life and food correctly and confidently, is based on knowing what's happening *right now,* and the only way to know, is to *be all there* right now.

The experience of the past is a secondary and inferior consideration. The past is academic; the present is real life, lived in real time. It's whole and complete so is free of error, uncertainty, and the need to overeat. A rule of thumb is this: When anxious, you're in the future; when depressed, you're in the past. When you're not present, you're in doubt, fear and error. When present, you're living from your higher subconscious mind, the foundation of all clarity, confidence and appetite-controlling knowledge and power.

The Present is The Point of Food Freedom

All of our thinking and feeling happens in and out of the present; and in order for the mind to be responsive to what's happening outside of it, it must be *flexible and free.* The more free, the more adaptable to lightning-fast, moment-to-moment activity. In order for awareness to keep up, it must move at the same speed as reality, and paradoxically, the only way it can do that is to remain perfectly relaxed and responsive. Thus there's no time or space for past conditioning to inveigle itself into your stomach.

The present is equal to the meditation state, when your attention is focused at the intersection of consciousness in order to notice the slightest movement. Mental stillness and presence of mind are one and the same state. As soon as the mind leaves stillness to become emotional – you've left the moment as well. The rule of thumb is this: If your mind is still, you are here; if it's going, you are gone. *To maintain the present moment, just maintain your detached, witnessing mindset.* It's virtually impossible to overeat in the present moment because the inherent power of the present neutralizes any unwanted desire or habit.

The present moment and the stress-free state of

detachment are the same. The present is like neutral gear in an automobile, the position in which there's no "stress" on the engine, and the position in which the car is now poised to move in any direction at any time. The future and past are like the forward and reverse gears; they are the positions of movement or emotion. In the forward position you can't go backwards; and in reverse you can't go forward. So you're not only stressed, but limited to only one position at a time. To choose one position is to sacrifice the other. In any given moment, half your potential is denied. But in present-moment reality, you can move in neutral, forward and reverse, all at the same time.

How? Because emotional movement and creative movement work in different directions: Emotional movement is toward the future or the past; but creative movement is inward and outward. By conceiving inwardly and expressing it outwardly, you're not only able to travel in "neutral" and without stress, but you can travel in both forward and reverse at the same time as well – for as you move, you pull the entire past and the entire future along with you at the same time. When you move in the right direction, the whole subconscious universe, all knowledge, moves with you.

Recovering Common Sense

You want to live and eat spontaneously, by common sense and intuition – as if you never really lived before nor tasted food before. Freedom is living in accordance with how things *really* are, not with how you *think* they are. Thinking takes time but life is instantaneous. Thinking is living around life, not in and to life. In order to be sensitive and receptive to the ever-changing newness of it, the old must be continually dropped. We cannot write on a chalkboard filled with yesterday's scribbles; it must first be erased. Otherwise the past will not only influence, affect and interfere with the present, it'll *prevent* the present as well. If you want something, you have to make a space for it.

Freedom is direct and immediate knowing and responding. It's a state of total flexibility and open-mindedness where there's no time or space between what's happening and a response that's appropriate to it. You are connected to the moment as directly and harmoniously as a dancer to his partner. When he moves forward, she simultaneously moves backwards, and vice versa. Their movements are not thought about or premeditated, and exactly *because* they're not, a perfect synchrony is automatically and effortlessly maintained. They've acquired "muscle memory" and have let go of mental memory. That's what you want to do: acquire "detachment memory" in order to maintain transcendence over your eating-for-comfort memory.

Ending Hangovers

To live from the past is like suffering a permanent hangover. When we eat or drink too much, the next day is affected. Instead of waking to a new day refreshed and alert, the mind and body remain dull and heavy. We're not free to relax and enjoy today because of yesterday's residue. Yesterday is no longer real or relevant but merely a concept, a memory. To have our lives controlled and determined by the past is a denial of the present – which is a denial of reality itself. As physical hangovers are of the past so are psychological and emotional hangovers. We overeat because we think that's just the way we are. We lived in our program and didn't know it like a fish lives in water and doesn't know it.

Each moment is unique as a fingerprint. You're not the same person you were a moment ago and if alive, won't be the same person a moment from now either. The experience of this moment will change you so that you'll act and respond in a new and different way in the next moment. This is true freedom, and attachment to anything whatsoever – especially to food, is the very killer of it.

There are no good or bad experiences as far as neutral awareness is concerned; there are only different and changing experiences, like clouds passing in the sky. The nature of reality is constant change and growth. Change is the only thing permanent in life. Heraclitus said, "You cannot step in the same river twice." To cling to the taste of past pleasures is a denial of present-moment life, growth and reality. Each moment is a different snowflake, a different miracle. Carbon copies cannot exist among that which is alive but only with things that are dead. Only the dead are the same yesterday, today and tomorrow; the living are always moving, growing, creating.

Attaching To The Past

The person who clings to the past is like a cartoon character working on an assembly line in a bottling factory. If he doesn't move along at the speed of the conveyor belt, he'll miss a bottle, and when trying to catch it, the next one crashes to the floor, and when he tries to save it the next one falls, then the next, and the next. Or it's like a clerk in a doughnut shop who doesn't rotate the doughnuts properly: He always puts the fresh ones in back and leaves the stale ones in front, so customers always get the stale ones, never the fresh ones.

Life is always fresh, but becomes stale when we live in the past or the future. We cannot cling to anything in life because it's happening too fast, and we can't escape anything either because it's part of the landscape. The only choice remaining is to let go and flow along with it. Be indifferent to it. And in that holy indifference lies the relaxation and appetite-control we had been searching for all along. When the dog finally becomes frustrated and exhausted enough from chasing his own tail, he lies down in surrender – only to find his tail brushing against his lips.

Living with a Passion

If at any given moment, most of your attention is directed either toward the past or toward some future event or result – like your weight loss goal, then less energy and intelligence remains to facilitate achieving that goal. If you have one eye on the future, you'll have only one eye left with which to live in the goal. Living in the goal instead of the future is to already be there. This principle applies to your moment- to-moment goals as well as to long term goals. The present is both the point of desire and the point of attainment. If you're not present you'll miss it.

The moment at hand is the entrance to life and truth. Our task is to enter this moment and to realize and accept that there's no end to it. It's eternal and unlimited. When Robin Hood's opponent hit the bull's-eye, everyone "believed" the game was over and began to leave. But Robin Hood didn't believe it – and proceeded to split the arrow. This moment is like the arrow at the center of the bull's-eye – it can be split indefinitely. To the degree you remain in the center of the moment, the center of your goal, there's no end to the game; to the degree you look forward or backward, the game's over.

We Repeat What We Don't Repair

The idea is to experience this moment so completely that nothing of it is left over to carry and weigh you down. You want to enter the moment cleanly and leave it cleanly. End the moment when the moment is ended, not leave it with unresolved questions or hangovers of resentment, doubt, regret, guilt.

Let what comes up in the moment go down with it. Have no unfinished business. Find your house clean and leave it clean. Settle an issue on the spot. If the bully of temptation and craving isn't stood up to there and then, it will trouble you always. Make all your actions complete and total. A sharpshooter doesn't aim, *then* fires, he aims and fires simultaneously. There's no space between the aiming and the firing; it's a single, unified action. Let the moment be the same – single, unified, all-inclusive. Let it come out of itself and return to itself.

Penetrate each moment with calmness and contentment and leave it the same way – without accumulating anything in the process, such as the desire that the next moment be the same or different. To the degree you remain in the present, all the knowledge necessary to overcome any eating issue will be spontaneously available to you.

You are being constantly guided by an inner, subconscious sense or spirit of wholeness. This spirit or intuition tells you what course of action to take in all circumstances, what to say and not to say, what to do and when to do it, what to eat and when to stop eating. This harmonizing spirit wants you and your goals to become one happy whole. In present-moment detachment you become receptive to its direction and empowered to fulfill it. You become guided from within.

Degrees of Detachment

Detachment can come by degree, or all at once. You can gradually come to it over weeks or months; or, in a single spontaneous let-go, decades of mental and emotion attachments, baggage and false beliefs can drop in a flash. The instant route is, of course, more appealing, but spontaneity cannot be premeditated; it's an obvious contradiction. You'll either become spontaneously detached or you won't, but you can't plan it. What you can do, however, is stay ready and receptive so that, in the first place, it *can* come, and in the second place, when it does, you'll *be there*. You want to at least be always in the ballpark.

The nature of spontaneity is to delight by surprise, but if you're never home, or the doors and windows of your mind are closed, you'll keep missing and missing. It's like the door-to-door salesman who needs only one sale per day to earn a living, but in order to make that one sale, he must knock on fifty doors. And just as the salesman can't know in advance which house contains the buyer, you can't know at which moment unprecedented degrees of Detachment will come, but you have to remain ready, alert and receptive at *every* moment.

The present is elusive and precarious. Once you've found it, you have to hang onto it like a surfer riding the crest of a wave. The crest is his "moment." Once he's found it, he can't let it go. While riding it, he's in heaven and the very picture of grace and beauty. But if he loses it – into the sea he flops.

Or it's like a rodeo cowboy riding a bucking bronco. Sitting on the bull when the bell rings and the gate swings open is the rider's *moment*. As long as he and the bull move as one animal, all's well; nothing negative can happen to him. But as soon as a little time or space develops between the bull's back and the cowboy's bottom – that's the end of the cowboy.

Surrendering To The Moment

The way to be free is to give up your ego to the present moment, to risk everything in it, put all your trust in it. What have you to lose but your excess mental, emotional and physical weight. Before there can be the new mind-body, the old has to be dropped. Before you can awaken, past programs have to be put to sleep. Health, happiness and freedom demand that nothing be held back. Commitment has to be total and constant. There can be no looking back, no doubt, fear or hesitation, for this moment is all there is, all there ever has been, all there ever will be or needs to be. Within it is realized the whole theme of existence – to relax and enjoy your beautiful new life, mind and body.

Key Points and Principles:

1. That present-moment centeredness is achieved by remaining consciously detached from the past and the future.

2. That the present moment nullifies all past habits and conditioning.

3. That the present moment is the point of the 6C's: Calmness, Contentment, Clarity, Control, Centeredness and Confidence.

4. That the present transcends emotional conflict.

5. That the present overcomes temptation and craving.

6. That the present is the point of comfort, security and power.

7. That the present is the point of flexibility, spontaneity and freedom.

8. That depression is of the past and anxiety is of the future.

9. That being present is about maintaining a detached, witnessing mindset.

10. That the present is the central guidance and reference point of clarity and appetite-control power.

APPENDIX 1

The Overeating Habit
BOOK SYNOPSIS

THE HABIT AND THE REMEDY

1. You've Acquired The Habit of Eating For Emotional Comfort Instead of Physical Nourishment;

2. This Wrong Purpose & Relationship Prevents You From Controlling Your Appetite;

3. You Correct The Relationship With Yourself & Food By Thinking, Feeling & Eating From A Conscious *Distance* Instead of From Emotional Involvement!

I. THE HABIT-BREAKING METHOD
    A. Eat *slowly & detachedly*, while
    B. Watching for the *exact point* the hunger abates,
    C. Then *stop* eating immediately!

II. PLANNING TO EAT, EATING TO PLAN
    A. *Pre-plan* 5 meals a day with nothing in between.
    B. *Weigh & measure* all meals (Weight-losing phase).
    C. *Record* all meals to maintain due diligence.

III. REVISING YOUR SELF-IMAGE
    A. Mind-body change is *predicated* on self-image.
    B. Change self-image by *convincing* the subconscious.
    C. Your prime motivation is freedom & self-control.

IV. VISUALIZING YOUR FUTURE
    A. *Vividly* picture yourself at your goal weight & size.
    B. Hold the attitude that you're *already* there.
    C. Feel the joy & satisfaction *now* that you'll feel then.

V. MOVING YOUR BODY
    A. Physical & Recreational Activities.
    B. Flexibility & Strength Exercises.
    C. Aerobic Activities.

VI. CONTROLLING YOUR EMOTIONS
    A. Experience the negative & positive with equanimity
    B. Be *above* all thought, feeling, desire & action.
    C. Don't be affected by one thing more than another .

VII. KEEPING YOUR DISTANCE
    A. *Detachment* is primary method of appetite control.
    B. *Detachment* is method of being centered, balanced.
    C. *Detachment* is method of unprecedented clarity.

VIII. OVERCOMING YOUR STRESS
    A. Stress is the primary trigger & fuel for overeating.
    B. The *emotional* pursuit of pleasure causes stress.
    C. The stress-free you are *above* all experience.

IX. TAKING LIFE IMPERSONALLY
    A. Act according to *role*, not thought or feeling.
    B. Let the *situation* determine your role & behavior.
    C. "*Service*" is the principle of successful relationship.

X. SEIZING THE MOMENT
    A. The *present* is the point of appetite-control.
    B. The *present* is above all inner & outer experience.
    C. The *present* reveals error, overcomes negativity.

APPENDIX 2 – BMI CHART (Body Mass Index)

BMI is a measurement of body fat based on height and weight that applies to both men and women between the ages of 18 and 65 years. BMI can be used to indicate if you are overweight, obese, underweight or normal. A healthy BMI score is between 19 and 24. A value from 25 to 29 indicates you may be overweight. Over 30 means you may be obese.

Height in Inches/Body Weight in Pounds

BMI	19	20	21	22	23	24	25	26	27	28	29	30	31	32	33
58	91	96	100	105	110	115	119	124	129	134	138	143	148	153	158
59	94	99	104	109	114	119	124	128	133	138	143	148	153	158	163
60	97	102	107	112	118	123	128	133	138	143	148	153	158	163	168
61	100	106	111	116	122	127	132	137	143	148	153	158	164	169	174
62	104	109	115	120	126	131	136	142	147	153	158	164	169	175	180
63	107	113	118	124	130	135	141	146	152	158	163	169	175	180	186
64	110	116	122	128	134	140	145	151	157	163	169	174	180	186	192
65	114	120	126	132	138	144	150	156	162	168	174	180	186	192	198
66	118	124	130	136	142	148	155	161	167	173	179	186	192	198	204
67	121	127	134	140	146	153	159	166	172	178	185	191	198	204	211
68	125	131	138	144	151	158	164	171	177	184	190	197	203	210	216
69	128	135	142	149	155	162	169	176	182	189	196	203	209	216	223
70	132	139	146	153	160	167	174	181	188	195	202	209	216	222	229
71	136	143	150	157	165	172	179	186	193	200	208	215	222	229	236
72	140	147	154	162	169	177	184	191	199	206	213	221	228	235	242
73	144	151	159	166	174	182	189	197	204	212	219	227	235	242	250
74	148	155	163	171	179	186	194	202	210	218	225	233	241	249	256
75	152	160	168	176	184	192	200	208	216	224	232	240	248	256	264
76	156	164	172	180	189	197	205	213	221	230	238	246	254	263	271

Source: U.S. Department of Health & Human Services. This chart is a general guide & won't apply to everyone. It doesn't take into account different body frames, muscle tone, etc. If not sure, consult a health-care professional as to the appropriate target weight for you.

ABOUT THE AUTHOR

My formal training was in electronics engineering, a field I abandoned after a certain "spiritual awakening" experience led me to an intense, 30-year study of human potential development. I researched comparative religion, philosophy and psychology with Eastern and Western teachers, gurus and mystics worldwide, and learned that what I'd discovered and directly experienced was the *Law of Detachment!*

It happened in 1976, quite accidentally and dramatically. I was a young electronics prodigy working at Lab for Electronics in Natick, Massachusetts, on a secret, aircraft navigation system for the U.S. Air Force. My job was to design an integrated circuit through which high frequency radio waves could pass with minimal resistance.

I succeeded in designing a perfectly "balanced" circuit in which the friction or resistance was virtually immeasurable. The circuit was, in effect, invisible, allowing radio waves to flow at maximum efficiency. I then saw a correlation between this phenomenon and how the mind works: In a balanced circuit there's no resistance; in a balanced mind there must also be no resistance, no blockage, no limitation. Mind, body and spirit must connect, unify, integrate.

With this revelation, my awareness spontaneously "detached" from the thoughts, feelings and activities that I was aware of. I drew back to a position of being neutral or centered – between my personal self and my aware or "spiritual" self. This backward movement extricated my awareness from its entanglement with the lower mental, emotional and sensual faculties.

I became both a witness to life and a participant at the same time. I was at once on the outside looking in and the inside looking out. I could see people, places and situations as they really are rather than as I thought, felt or believed they are.

I experienced the definition of reality to be – that which exists before we personalize it. In other words, the whole secret of life is to not take anything personally, and is achieved by "keeping a distance" from all internal and external experience.

This unprecedented ability to see from a distance was a virtual heaven-on-earth experience – too wonderful for words to describe; so joyful, enlightening and empowering, that all the rest of life became worthless in comparison, and I've devoted my life to the continued study, practice and teaching of it.

Bill is a meditation and hypnosis expert, a spiritual teacher specializing in the law of detachment, and a life coach specializing in weight management. He lives in Naples, Florida and spends his semi-retirement coaching a highly-rated, one-on-one, 30-day program on The Overeating Habit – based on this book. The private program is presented live locally or via Skype, internationally.

Visit his website at CoachMcLaughlin.com
Write him at: Info@CoachMcLaughlin.com